Step-by-Step Guide to Foraging Edible Wild Plants

The 38 Mountain West Plants You Need to Know

Kami Kessel

Table of Contents

CHAPTER 6: SHROOMIN' AROUND 111

CHAPTER 7: NATURAL MEDICINE 136

Introduction

I'm going to give you a handful of wild flowers, so each petal that falls will remind you that the earth breathes, and the moon rises.
–Carolyn Riker

Do you feel out of sorts thinking about spending another day at the mall or online? Instead, would you like to head outdoors and get some fresh air and sunshine? Would you also want to do something productive and useful with your time while enjoying the great outdoors? Have you wondered whether the different plants, berries, or fruits you come across in the wild are edible? How amazing would it be if you could come home with a basket full of delicious goodness of 100% natural ingredients whenever you spend some time outdoors? Does this sound appealing to you? If yes, you might start foraging.

Foraging is the simple act of identifying and gathering foods in the wild. This is not a new concept, and humans have been foraging since time immemorial. However, modernization of the world has widened the gap between us and nature. If you are tired of life's complexities, want a break from consumeristic living, and want to reconnect with nature, then foraging is an excellent means to achieve these goals. Foraging can help supplement your diet with delicious, wild edibles that don't cost you a penny and are yours for the taking. This is a great way to increase the nutrient content of the food you eat without increasing the grocery bills. You can do this while learning more about the local ecosystem of the region where you live or are planning to visit — the Mountain West.

One of the largest and most diverse regions within the United States is the Mountain West, also known as the Mountain States. It includes New Mexico, Colorado, Wyoming, Utah, Nevada, Arizona, Montana, and Idaho, from the High Plains to the Sierra Nevada and the Cascade Range. The terrain of the Mountain West is also more diverse than any other region within the United States. Its physical geography includes some of the highest mountain peaks in the continental United States, plus rolling, wide open plains in the eastern portion of this region, and even desert lands. One word that aptly describes the geography of this region is diverse.

The more diverse the terrain, the greater the variety of plants found in the region. This is one of the reasons why the Mountain West is one of the best regions to forage wild edible plants. It bears stating the obvious: not everything that you see in the wild is edible. Also, just because some berries look delicious or some seeds resemble something you have previously eaten, you cannot assume that they are edible. Therefore, you must learn thoroughly to identify edible wild foods before attempting to eat wild foods. The good news is that you have found a good resource here in this book to start to learn about gathering wild foods. The information provided in this book needs to be used together with other reliable sources and cannot be exclusively relied upon to determine whether what you find in the wild is edible. There are many dangerous plants and mushrooms that look very similar to edible varieties, and therefore, unless you are 100% positive that it is safe to eat, do not ingest or handle.

As you gain knowledge about edible wild plants, you can also make the most of the different benefits foraging offers. From encouraging you to spend more time outdoors and reconnecting with nature to becoming environmentally conscious and breathing in the fresh air, foraging is a brilliant physical and mental activity. All of this may reduce stress and improve the overall quality of your life, too. Also, foraging adventures can become a means to detox from the hustle and bustle of city life while helping you to get back to your roots.

Are you wondering how I've learned all this? I believe it is time for a little introduction. Hello, my name is Kami Kessel, and I'm a yoga teacher, yoga therapist, and certified health and wellbeing coach. I grew up riding horses bareback with my cousins in Conifer, Colorado. I was a part of 4H and Girl Scouts from childhood, and these experiences stayed with me as I transitioned into adulthood. I was a Girl Scouts Leader and First-Aider for more than 15 years. I not only understand how helpful nature is, but I also know first-hand the basics of how to be prepared and enjoy safe adventures in nature. Many people feel disconnected from nature, and I love helping people reconnect with their roots and fall back in love with the beautiful outdoors. In this book I have gathered information from regional sources to help you along your path in beginning to learn about the many benefits of foraging. Exploring the outdoors and foraging for lovely foods can bring enjoyment and well-being into your life in unexpected ways and leave you pleasantly surprised. Also, being in nature itself can be a terrific healer. So, maybe it is time to try and get in touch with it.

In this book you will learn about what foraging means, tips and steps to become an ethical forager, and some legal and safety protocols to remember. Please note that I am not providing any legal advice, but am happy to share my findings on many of the requirements that may apply. It is up to you to determine what specific regulations may apply to your specific foraging, both by geographic location and substance. Once you learn the basics, you will be introduced to different types of edible nuts and seeds found in the wild and begin to learn how to identify them, delicious roots and tubers commonly found in the Mountain West, and ultimately how to harvest them. You will also learn about a variety of wild greens that are not only edible but incredibly delicious and filled with a variety of nutrients. You will learn about the juicy goodness of fruits and berries found in this region. You will also be introduced to various edible mushrooms commonly found in the Mountain West, along with their identifying factors. Apart from this, you will discover a list of medicinal herbs commonly used to treat different ailments and tips to recognize them.

So, this book will act as a guide for nearly every step of the way. Before you decide to head outdoors and start foraging, it is crucial that you spend the needed time to carefully go through the details in this book along with additional resources and work with a local expert to ensure that you are correctly applying the information learned. While learning to identify plants in the wild, it is crucial that you never rely on a single factor or a single resource. Instead, you need to focus on multiple factors for proper identification. Without this, the chances of accidentally misidentifying a plant are quite high. Don't be in a rush. A steep learning curve is involved in foraging. However, your efforts will certainly be worth it once you gain the level of confidence and knowledge to start harvesting delicious and nutritious ingredients in the Mountain West.

Nature offers a wide variety of edible plants to forage, provided you know where to look. When it comes to foraging, you should not only focus on gathering wild foods; learning to enjoy them is also important. After all, your time, energy, and effort went into this process. Therefore, learning to honor and enjoy the items foraged is needed, too. Are you wondering how you can do this? All that it requires is a little creativity and a willingness to experiment with different ingredients in the kitchen. In this book you can also discover simple and delicious recipes using the wild ingredients discussed. Simply gather the needed ingredients and follow the steps, and voila, a meal is ready within no time. Once you get the hang of different flavor combinations that work, don't hesitate to experiment a little!

This book will not only help you to reconnect with nature, and become more conscious of how you can help it, but it will also show how foraging can be a part of sustainable living. Foraging also allows you to explore areas and interact more with nature. Combining these factors may possibly improve the overall quality of your life.

Are you eager to learn more about foraging? Do you want to discover the nutritious and delicious treasures in the Mountain West? If yes, let's get started!

Chapter 1:

Before You Go

Resilience is all about being able to overcome the unexpected.
Sustainability is about survival. The goal of resilience is to thrive.
–Jamais Cascio

Humans have relied on nature for their survival since the dawn of civilization. From the beginning, our ancestors depended on whatever was available to them to obtain the sustenance needed to survive. However, long gone are those days when foraging was a means of survival. Instead, these days, it has become a well-loved activity that is rapidly gaining popularity. It is quite likely that you might have foraged at some point but didn't realize it was called foraging. Whether it is picking berries from a nearby park or a day spent in the local woods looking for edible leaves, these are instances of foraging.

So, what is foraging? The simple act of gathering food in the wild is termed foraging. It involves actively searching, identifying, and collecting food resources found in the wild. Whether it's herbs, fruits, mushrooms, plants, or flowers, different things grow in nature without human interference. There is plenty available in nature, provided you know what you are looking for and where to look for it. Foraging has also been gaining popularity for different reasons ranging from reduction in carbon footprint to better understanding of the ecosystem and adopting an environmentally conscious lifestyle. It is also a great excuse to get away from the hustle and bustle of city life and spend some time reconnecting with your roots in nature.

Foraging probably sounds quite simple. How hard can it be to collect food in the wild? You need to grab a basket and pluck all the ingredients you come across, don't you? Well, not exactly. Foraging involves a steep learning curve. Even though plenty of edible plants are found in the wild, there are several poisonous ones too, and as foraging experts will tell you, one nibble can kill.

Some plants very closely resemble their edible counterparts but are incredibly harmful to humans. Therefore, you need to be extremely safe while foraging. In this chapter, you will be introduced to different safety tips and precautions that will help you learn how to forage ethically and safely in the wild outdoors. Please remember, if you are not 100% positive that it is safe to eat, do not ingest or handle your findings.

Stay Safe While Foraging

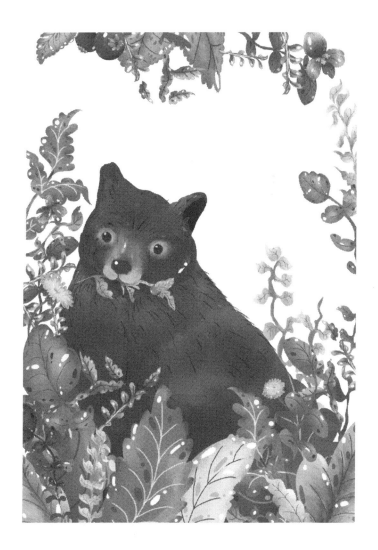

Maybe you've seen jokes in online foraging forums to go "au naturel" when you forage. I know I have seen these jokes, and I hope they are jokes, although I don't find them all that funny. The truth is, it's quite important to wear and bring appropriate equipment with you. While there is risk associated with any activity, especially in the wild, we can prepare ourselves for success with knowledge, planning, and appropriate caution.

When you head out to forage, wear long pants, long sleeves, and a hat. Tuck your pants into thick socks and wear sturdy boots with ankle support. Tuck your sleeves into thick gloves. Wear a bandana around your neck and make sure the neck opening of your shirt is covered. Use bug spray at each of these junction points and carefully check yourself for ticks after you've returned from foraging. If you don't want to use bug spray, consider draping mosquito netting over a wide brimmed hat and tucking this into your neckline under the bandana. Wear broad-spectrum sunscreen of at least SFP 30 on any exposed areas.

Bring as much water to drink as you can carry, and if you will be out for more than one day, bring a water filter method. You can research water filtration on your own if you need to.

Also, learn about and be prepared for any encounters with wildlife that are relevant to where you are headed. Tell friends or family specifically where you are going, and for how long. Make a plan for check-ins with

start with taking photos and notes. Then, as you begin to learn important tools, decide when you feel it is appropriate to begin handling wild plants.

Ethical Foraging

When it comes to foraging, you should not only pay attention to what you can forage but should learn about all that you need to avoid, for your own safety, and also to preserve nature. That is, enjoy nature's bounty without destroying it or harming yourself. This is what the concept of ethical foraging is all about. You must forage so that it is sustainable for other foragers, wildlife, and the future. In your excitement, avoid the tendency to be greedy, and don't harvest everything you see. Remember that nature is not an all-you-can-eat buffet that exists to solely serve your needs and requirements.

One of the simplest ways to become an ethical forager is to avoid picking all plant parts. Avoid foraging more than one-third of a plant at any given point. Also, harvest only what is needed. For instance, if you know that you will only use the leaves or fruits of a specific plant, uprooting it is a bad idea. Before you harvest a plant, follow the native Cherokee rule of four. This means a plant must be harvested only if you pass by that particular variety at least four times. This ensures there is plenty of the specific plant, and you aren't endangering it. Always be conservative in your harvests. Avoid harvesting the entire plant if you know you will not be using it. Likewise, if a plant seems to be in short supply, don't harvest it. For instance, if you notice only a single patch of a specific plant and don't come across more of it, stay away from it. This is a great rule to follow and helps reduce the risk of accidentally harvesting an endangered or at-risk species. Also, rotate your foraging areas. This gives the plants a chance to regrow and so they can be foraged later. If you have harvested a specific plant from a spot, avoid foraging from the same spot immediately. Instead, give nature a while to grow and develop again.

If you notice that any roots are dislodged, replant them. Similarly, you can also scatter seeds of certain plants to promote their growth. Learning to be an ethical forager is one of the best ways to ensure that you aren't damaging the environment. Always leave the area you have foraged from in an undisturbed condition as much as possible. For instance, instead of twisting off a plant's stem, it is better to clip a twig or snip the leaves to ensure the plant can heal and grow. By following ethical foraging practices, you can strengthen your bond with nature. It will also teach you the importance of respecting and caring for the local ecosystem. So, avoid altering the local landscape. After all, it isn't just you that depends on nature. There are others, too, including the local wildlife.

Rules and Legal Guidelines

Rules and regulations are prevalent in all aspects of life. They are set in place to ensure your safety and that of others. Not following the said rules could land you in legal trouble. After all, not being aware of the law is not a permissible excuse. To become an ethical forager, you must learn about the local rules and guidelines associated with foraging. The rules about foraging in public areas differ from one region to another. The Mountain West region is quite vast and covers different states. So, carefully check state and county regulations about foraging before you head out.

For instance, in most areas, there is a list of plants considered at-risk or endangered. Foraging such plants will attract trouble through penalties and fines. Similarly, there are often quantity limits on how much of a plant can be harvested. For instance, per the mushroom foraging laws in Utah, no permit is needed to harvest mushrooms for personal use, but there is a limit on the number of mushrooms that can be harvested. The law prohibits harvesting more than 10 pounds of mushrooms per person for personal use. A permit is needed if you wish to harvest more than this limit. In Idaho, there isn't a restriction on the recreational picking of berries found in the wild; however, there are limits on the amount that can be collected.

Per the electronic code of federal regulations for US National Parks, there is a strict prohibition against destroying, injuring, defacing, digging, or removing something from its natural habitat. Certain limits are enforced about the size and quantity of natural products that can be gathered. Gathering any natural foods beyond the permissible limits is a punishable offense. In some areas, foraging isn't allowed at all without a permit.

Along the same lines, the chances of accidentally trespassing cannot be overlooked. When out in the wild, it can be quite tricky to determine where public property ends and private property begins. Therefore, you need to be extremely careful about where you forage. If not, you might unknowingly end up in legal trouble. After all, which private property owner would be happy when someone trespasses on their property or others are helping themselves to the food they're growing? This is why you need to carefully check the regulations regarding the chosen foraging area. Also check whether the said area is tribal land or property.

The simplest way to take care of this step is to check with the local wildlife authorities. Usually, you will notice signposts about the activities that aren't allowed in a region. If any permits are needed, get them. You can often forage on private lands, provided you have a permit for it. If not, you are trespassing, which is a criminal offense, and you can be penalized. Depending on where you are foraging or wish to forage, the laws and regulations change. So, consider foraging with local foragers or an expert to get a better sense of what to do and avoid. This is also a reason you must always carry a map of the region you are foraging in.

Keeping all these requirements in mind, one of the most important things you must remember about foraging is that there is plenty that you can obtain from nature. Different herbs and greens are commonly found throughout the Mountain West region. Chances are you have come across many of these plants but never knew they were edible!

Chapter 2:

Ah Nuts

Seeds and nuts are indispensable for cardiovascular health. The protective properties of nuts against coronary heart disease were first recognized in the early 1990s, and a strong body of literature has followed, confirming these original findings. –Joel Fuhrman

Incorporating nuts and seeds into your daily diet can be a wonderful idea and can improve your overall health and ensure that your body gets its daily dose of nutrition. Nuts and seeds are an incredible source of protein, fiber, healthy and desirable fats, and a variety of vitamins and minerals. There are different types of nuts and seeds that can be easily incorporated into any diet. They can enrich lots of recipes, and on their own nuts and seeds make for an excellent snack. They can be used as garnish, butter can be made with nuts and seeds, and they can be used in desserts, too. Nuts and seeds are truly versatile and offer a variety of health benefits.

Nuts are considered an extremely good source of heart-healthy fats, contain plenty of protein, and have compounds that can maintain the health of blood vessels. They are also free of cholesterol and have high levels of fiber. They also have different vitamins and minerals, such as vitamin B6, niacin, magnesium, calcium, zinc, selenium, potassium, phosphorus, and other antioxidants. Seeds have a similar nutritional profile. Both nuts and seeds can also help our bodies absorb nutrients from foods such as greens.

Things to Remember

If you are foraging anything in the wild, ensure that you do it ethically, which is incredibly important with nuts and seeds. Do not only focus on satisfying your immediate needs but preserve enough for future harvests and for wildlife, who depend on these nutritional powerhouses. That said, you can sustainably harvest nuts and seeds. It's also important to know what you must do to enjoy the nuts and seeds. For instance, acorns harvested from an oak tree are usually bitter due to tannins present in them. Therefore, a dedicated process is needed to make them palatable. On the other hand, shagbark hickory nuts are already tender and sweet, so you simply need to crack the outer shell and eat the nut. Similarly, black walnuts taste incredibly good, but separating the nut from the fruit and shell can be an elaborate process. So, be sure to bring with you a nutcracker to crack the shell of most nuts, such as hazelnuts, butternuts, and black walnuts, plus a pair of scissors or pruners and a cloth or paper bag.

Look for nuts and seeds in semi-forested areas, marshlands, and areas next to creeks and rivers. Nuts are also found in dense forests. Opt for fruit that is ready to let go from the tree. When the fruits are ripe, shake the tree and collect everything that has fallen to the ground. Alternatively, you can also cut the fruit away from the tree. Similarly, to harvest seeds, clip seed heads off at the stem or prune using sharp pruners.

The ideal season to look for nuts is fall and winter because the plants drop their fruit at this time (and hurry, because the local wildlife will also be excited to feast on them). The best season to look for seeds is late summer. That said, there are variations in these seasonal guidelines. For instance, hazelnuts ripen quicker than most nuts, and you need not wait until mid-fall to harvest them.

Common Nuts and Seeds to Look For

You might be excited to start foraging nuts and seeds after learning about the benefits they offer. Please remember the above-mentioned suggestions about things to remember while foraging nuts and seeds. Let's look at common nuts and seeds found in the Mountain West. You will learn to identify them along with the different benefits they offer.

Hazelnuts

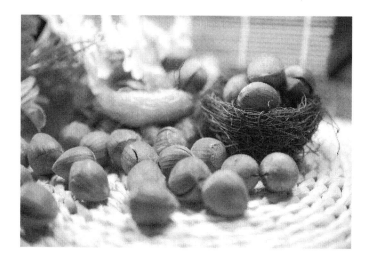

A variety of species of trees belong to the hazel family, most of which produce edible nuts. Hazelnut trees are rather large shrubs that belong to the Corylus genus. Around 14-18 known hazel species are commonly placed in the Betulaceae plant family, which includes birch trees. So, it is safe to say that hazels are related to birch trees! Hazelnut trees are usually believed to be native to the temperate northern hemisphere and are commonly known for the nuts they produce.

The most common type of hazelnut tree in the United States is the beaked hazelnut. This deciduous shrub is native to North America. When fully mature, it can be between four and eight meters tall. Its stems are easily distinguishable because of their smooth and gray-colored bark. The leaves themselves are oval or round and have double serrated margins. The leaves are slightly hairy on the underside. When fully mature, the leaves can be between five and 11 cm long and around three to eight centimeters wide.

Lovely flowers are produced by this tree. The nuts that follow are enclosed in a hull-like structure resembling a beak, hence their name. The nuts ripen between September and October. You'll need to be quick if you want to harvest these nuts because other animals love feasting on them, too!

These nuts can be eaten right off the tree or saved for later. When it comes to nuts, you will need to get rid of the external hull or the shell and then eat the kernel inside. Hazelnuts can be used just like any other nuts, in baking, cooking, or making a salad. You can also make hazelnut butter by grinding the nuts with or without sweetener.

Acorns

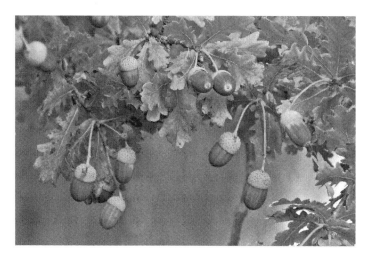

The fruit obtained from oak trees is known as acorns. Hundreds of species of acorns exist, and around 90 of them are native to the United States. Acorns are also among the easiest to identify and harvest. Speaking of easy to harvest, the oak tree next to our house literally "throws" acorns onto the ground during one week in late summer. Our wildlife friends harvest them very efficiently and they are gone in no time. Acorns are easy to store, too. Most species of acorns don't have any specific taste or flavor and are quite similar to wheat or even corn. Humans have been eating acorns since time immemorial. Assyrians and Greeks were known to eat acorns regularly due to their nutrient contents. Some Native American tribes regularly forage acorns in the wild even today.

Acorns contain various healthy fats, calcium, fiber, magnesium, phosphorus, potassium, and other nutrients. Heart-healthy Omega-3 fatty acids present in them, along with antioxidants, are considered to regulate blood cholesterol levels, improve cardiovascular function, and also help tackle inflammation.

So, how can you identify acorns? If you have live in the United States, chances are you know how to identify an oak tree. If you can identify an oak tree, you have found acorns too! The distinctive silhouette of the oak tree makes them fairly straightforward to identify. The trees usually have a wide and well-rounded canopy that takes up around two-thirds of their overall height. When mature, these trees are extremely tall. They also have a distinctive branch structure. The branches are thick and kinked, and it looks as if they grow without a straight leading stem. The branches grow alternatingly, and there is no opposing growth because the buds are arranged in a spiral fashion. This means branches grow randomly in all directions.

The bark of the young oak trees is irregular with shallow grooves and is grayish brown colored. The bark thickens with age but remains a darker shade of gray. The leaves make it quite easy to identify oak trees. The leaves are usually longer than wide and have five to seven leaves on each side. The leaves grow in a spiral pattern. Acorns are the shiny, ovoid fruits produced by oak trees. They have textured caps. Initially, they are green, and slowly take on their typical brown color with age.

There are multiple ways to use acorns. They can be eaten whole, turned into flour, or even used to extract oil. However, you will first need to remove the tannins in them. Tannins taste bitter, and when consumed in large amounts, are toxic. Tannins are anti-nutrients; when you consume tannins, your body is prevented from effectively obtaining nutrients from any food you consume. The good news is that these tannins can be removed from acorns. To do this, boil the acorns in water and wait until the water turns brown. After this, remove the water and restart the process. Keep doing this until the water no longer turns brown. At this stage, the acorns are ready for you to prepare and enjoy. Remove the acorns from the water, pat them dry, and then decide how you want to use them. Don't try eating the acorns without removing the tannins.

Black Walnuts

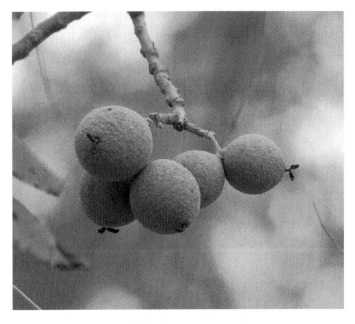

Did you know that walnut trees also grow in the wild? These delicious nuts can be easily foraged in the Mountain West region, provided you know what to look for. The ones that grow in the wild are commonly known as black walnuts. The scientific name of the black walnut tree is *Juglans nigra*, and it is a native hardwood tree found in specific Mountain West locations. Usually, in the area where black walnut trees are growing, you might not find other ground covers because they produce a chemical that hinders the growth of other trees around them.

Now, let's learn about identifying the black walnut tree, which can be up to 120 feet tall when fully mature. Their average height is around 80 feet tall. The trunk usually appears long because its first branches start high on the tree itself. Initially, the bark is gray and scaly when young; over time, it slowly darkens. It also develops diamond-shaped ridges. The leaves are also incredibly large and can be up to 24 inches long. The individual leaves are single leaflets and black walnut trees tend to be among the first to shed their leaves during autumn.

Another easy way to identify the black walnut trees is to look at their fruits. The tree starts dropping small tennis ball-sized fruit in September or October. The outer husk is initially yellow-green and turns black later. Gather the fruit you notice and try shaking more off the tree. This is the only means of harvesting the fruit. The next step is to extract the nut from it.

However, getting to the kernel or seed inside it is not an easy job. There are three parts to the fruit. It consists of a dry outer covering, which is known as the hull. Once you remove the hull, you will come across a hard shell. You need to crack this shell, and then you can get to the kernel. The kernel is that part of the walnut commonly eaten. You can also extract oil from it. The unique flavor and aroma of these nuts make an incredible addition to any dessert or baked goodies. Black walnuts are rich in minerals, fiber, and vitamin A. They are known to contain high levels of antioxidants and healthy fats.

Hickory Nuts

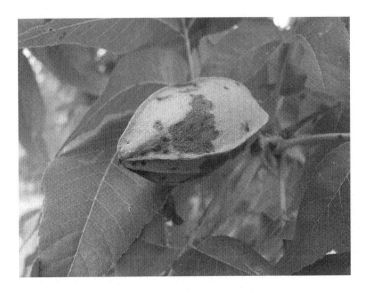

The fruit obtained from the hickory tree is known as hickory nuts. This tree belongs to the Carya genus. All types of hickory nuts are usually edible and taste quite similar to pecans. For that matter, did you know that the pecan is a type of hickory nut? Hickory nuts are usually classified as a specific type of nut-like drupe. This is because the hard shell splits open, revealing a softer fruit or seed in its center. As mentioned, there are different varieties of hickory nut trees; some taste quite bitter, while others are incredibly tasty.

You can eat the hickory nut right out of the shell and enjoy its delicious flavor. These nuts have double nutshells. The first layer is made of a greenish-brown husk that slowly dries as the nut matures. The outer husk turns brown as the nut is ready for harvest. This outer husk splits open to reveal a smooth, tough brown shell. Once you crack this shell, you can feast on the delicious hickory nut inside! This nutshell is slightly difficult to crack; therefore, always carry a nutcracker in your foraging kit.

Once you crack the tough outer shell, you can enjoy the sweet nuts on the inside. So, how do you identify hickory nuts? The first thing you need to do is identify the hickory tree. These trees have long compound leaves with large oblong leaflets that are lance-shaped. The leaves can be anywhere between 10 and 24 inches long. The peeling gray bark is another identifying factor of these trees. Apart from this, look for greenish-brown or brown husked fruits that are the same size as black walnuts.

Hickory trees can be found across the Mountain West region, especially in deciduous forests and woodlands. Collecting these nuts is a rather popular activity during the fall. Usually, hickory trees produce nuts yearly, but once every three years, the trees produce a bumper crop. Use them just like you would use pecans, and keep them in the freezer to prolong their shelf life.

Wild Millet Seeds

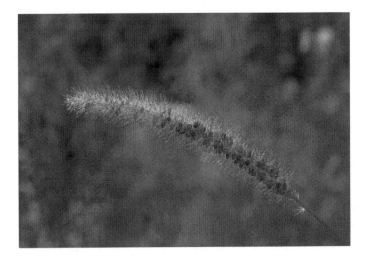

A variety of millets are found across the world. One of the most commonly found varieties of millets in the wild in the United States is the proso millet. It belongs to the grass family or Poaceae. The scientific name of this plant is *Panicum miliaceum*. This is an annual warm-weather-loving grass. It is commonly found across North America, including the Mountain West.

This plant can be nearly five feet tall when fully mature. This free-standing plant has an extremely shallow root system. This summer annual usually has branches close to its base, with simple alternating hairy leaves on each of its branches. The small fruit it produces is smooth and oblong, usually white to begin with but can also be found in different colors. The leaves themselves are long and oval-shaped and are a shade of light green.

You might also notice some lighter green spikes along the stem. You will find the seeds or grains consumed as cereals within these spikes. The seeds can be white or off-white, turning brown or black as they mature. To harvest millets, you simply need to snip the spikes with the seed-like structures.

To ensure all the stems are removed, you will need to clean the seedheads very well, because you consume only the tiny seeds. Once you have separated them, you have successfully harvested the edible seeds! You can add them to salads, or dry them and cook them like rice!

Amaranth Seeds

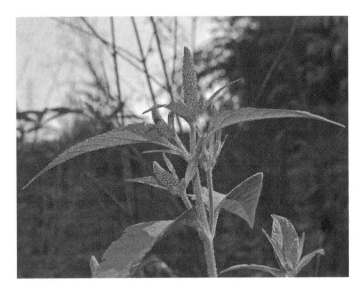

Amaranth is an ancient crop that is believed to have originated in the Americas. It's also used as a leafy vegetable when young, and the seeds produced are used just like any other grain. The species of green amaranth have been important to different cultures for thousands of years. Did you know that the Aztec civilization in Mexico during the 1400s had massive acreage dedicated to growing amaranth?

Amaranth belongs to the Amaranthus genus and includes more than 70 species. The most common variety of amaranth found in the Mountain West region is the Amaranthus palmeri. Here's an interesting fact about amaranth: it's related to the spinach family!

When fully mature, these plants can be up to seven feet tall. These broad-leaf plants have thick and tough stems that somewhat resemble sunflowers, and are slightly reddish in some varieties. The seeds are tiny and lens-shaped, and usually white or cream-colored. The seedheads can be very colorful. The plant sports very simple alternate leaves and tiny white flowers. The flower heads are conical and contain hundreds of seeds. The flower heads are usually green or red and slowly turn brown as they mature and dry out.

As mentioned, amaranth seeds can be used just like any other grain, including drying and then grinding into flour. The flour can then be used in cookies, bread, cakes, noodles, cereals, or other flour-based foods. Amaranth seeds are good sources of protein, filled with fiber, and low in saturated fats.

The young, tender plants can be cooked like any other leafy green, such as spinach, provided the stems and leaves aren't tough yet. The seeds are the most utilized part of the plant. Harvest the seed heads by snipping them at the base using sharp gardening shears. Collect all the tops and then dry them. Once dry, shake them, and the seeds will come apart. The seeds can be consumed directly from the plant or boiled later. The dried seeds can also be popped just like popcorn eaten as is, or used in baking.

Caraway Seeds

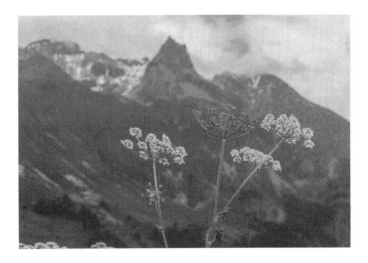

The scientific name of wild caraway is *Carum carvi*. This plant belongs to the parsley family and even resembles it to a certain extent. It is also referred to as Persian cumin and is believed to have originated as a flavoring used by ancient Arabic peoples. Even though it resembles cumin, its flavor profile is similar to that of star anise. This biennial plant sports flowers in the second year.

The seeds appear within a month of blooming, and then the plant starts to die. Since it is a self-seeding plant, a new one will soon regrow in its place. A wonderful thing about the caraway plant is it's not just the edible seeds; you can also consume their leaves and roots. The caraway seeds are unlike most others you will find.

The caraway plants usually prefer rocky terrain, and you can easily find them along the mountainous regions within the United States. Because of the plant's wavy shape and umbrels, it is commonly mistaken for wild parsley. Compared to other plants, caraway usually matures quite early in the season. These plants have extremely slender leaves and hollow stems. The umbrella-like clusters of small white flowers are surprisingly pretty. The alternate leaves are long and oblong.

When the plant is fully mature, it can be up to three feet tall and usually has one or more shoots that emerges from a single tap root system. The seeds produced by it are brown, narrow, and oblong. They resemble cumin but are slightly bigger and don't have the usual cumin-like aroma. Instead, the brown seeds with five distinct linear and tan ribs smell like star anise.

These seeds are a truly multifaceted spice and have also been used for medicinal purposes in Ayurveda and other systems. They contain fiber, copper, magnesium, manganese, iron, calcium, and various antioxidants.

Caraway seeds are used in baked goods such as dinner rolls, French toast, soda bread, muffins, and cookies. You can also add them to fruit-based desserts such as custards and jams. You can also feature them in savory recipes and chew on them after a meal. A fresh and calming herbal tea can be brewed with these seeds too.

Butternuts

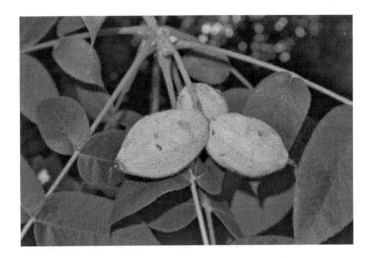

The scientific name of butternuts is *Juglans cinerea*. Butternuts are also referred to as white walnuts, and they are the sweet fruit obtained from the butternut tree. They resemble regular walnuts but don't have the characteristic bitterness associated with walnuts. Instead, butternuts taste quite similar to pine nuts and have a creamy and mild flavor.

Butternuts are incredibly versatile and can be incorporated into any dish that calls for walnuts or pine nuts. They are commonly found from mid-September until mid-October. So, if you stumble on football-shaped fruits in the wild, they might be butternuts. The outer layer of the fruit is covered in a fuzzy green husk with a smooth velvet-like texture. This layer is also slightly sticky and resinous. Press a finger against its surface, and it will stick to it! Butternuts also grow in clusters and fall off the tree as soon as they are ripe.

Their bark is rather distinctive; the ridged bark usually features raised portions with a silvery glint, followed by darker indentations. The ridges are always visible, even if the color contrast isn't dramatic. These ridges also form a distinctive diamond pattern. The alternate compound leaves culminate with a single leaflet at the tip. The leaves resemble those of a black walnut tree.

Once you gather the fruits, you must remove the husk to get to the delicious nut meat inside. A sharp paring knife will help score the husk and pop the outer layer.

Alternatively, you can use a rubber mallet to remove the outer husk. After this, the nuts need to be cured for a week, and then you can either consume them or store them for later. To cure them, line the nuts on trays and place them in a well-ventilated room for a couple of days. Keep rotating the nuts, so they dry evenly and don't mold. Once they are dry to touch, the nuts can be cracked open. A small rubber hammer or a nutcracker can then be used to break the shell and eat the nut. Use these nuts like walnuts and pecans.

Recipes

Here are some exciting and delicious recipes incorporating the nuts and seeds mentioned above that you foraged in the wild. Depending on the ingredients you (safely) forage, pick a recipe that strikes your fancy and get started!

A note about the recipes in this book: All of the recipes can be prepared vegan (that's what I do). The recipes are written to suit all types of eating styles but please customize as you want! For example, you can use non-dairy versions of ingredients and either substitute in a vegan version of something, or an equivalent amount of cooked lentils/beans with corresponding spices for any of the "meat" items mentioned.

Also, while a basic section about how to use commonly known herbs is included, please note that this guide focuses on foraging for foods to eat. Herbal medicine is a professional specialty that requires training beyond the scope of this guide.

Hazelnut Cookies

Serves: 20–25

Ingredients:

- 1 ⅓ cups skin-on hazelnuts
- ¼ teaspoon kosher salt
- 2 large egg whites
- 2/3 cup sugar

Directions:

1. Preheat the oven to 350° F.
2. Spread the hazelnuts on a baking sheet and toast in the preheated oven for about 12–15 minutes until golden brown.
3. Place the nuts on a kitchen towel. Gather the edges of the towel and cover the hazelnuts for about a minute.
4. Now rub the nuts well with the towel to remove skin, removing as much skin as possible. No issues if all the skin doesn't come off. Let the nuts cool to room temperature.
5. Turn down the temperature of the oven to 300° F.
6. Place the hazelnuts in a food processor and give short pulses until the nuts are coarsely chopped.
7. Add egg white and salt into a mixing bowl and beat with an electric hand mixer until stiff peaks are formed.
8. Add sugar and hazelnuts and fold gently until well incorporated.
9. Prepare a large baking sheet or use 2 baking sheets if required.
10. Drop a tablespoonful of the mixture on the baking sheet. Leave sufficient gaps between the cookies because they need a little air and also they spread a bit.
11. Place the baking sheet in the oven and set the timer for 15–18 minutes or until golden brown around the edges.

12. Let the cookies cool on the baking sheet for about 5–8 minutes. Cool completely on a wire rack.
13. Store in an airtight container. They can last up to 10 days refrigerated and longer in the freezer.

Acorn Ice Cream

Serves: 12–15

Ingredients:
- 4 cups heavy cream
- 6–8 tablespoons ground roasted acorns (acorn coffee)
- ¼ teaspoon salt
- 4 cups whole milk
- 12 egg yolks

Directions:
1. The acorns have to be prepared before using. Prepare the acorns by hot leaching the tannins from the acorns as I described in the chapter. Roast and grind the acorns.
2. Combine milk and ground acorns in a saucepan. Place the saucepan over medium-low heat. When the mixture just starts steaming, remove the saucepan from theat. Let it infuse for 20 minutes.

3. Place a fine mesh strainer over a bowl and pour the acorn milk into the strainer. Pour the strained milk into a clean saucepan.
4. Add yolks and cream into a bowl and whisk until well combined.
5. Pour yolk mixture into the saucepan with milk, a little at a time and whisk well each time.
6. When all of it is added, place the saucepan over low heat and whisk constantly until the temperature of the mixture is 170° F and it will start thickening and will coat the back of a spoon. Turn off the heat.
7. Transfer the milk mixture into a bowl. Cover the bowl with cling wrap such that it is touching the milk mixture, so that a "skin" doesn't form. Cool completely and chill for 5–6 hours.
8. Pour the mixture into an ice cream maker and churn the ice cream following the manufacturer's directions.

Hickory Nuts Shortbread Cookies

Serves: 15–18

Ingredients:
- ½ cup unsalted butter, softened
- ¼ teaspoon salt

- 6 tablespoons confectioners' sugar, sifted (be sure to sift!)
- ¼ cup finely chopped wild hickory nuts
- **⅛ teaspoon grated orange zest (optional)**
- 1 cup all-purpose flour
- ¼ teaspoon vanilla extract

Directions:

1. Place butter in the mixing bowl of the stand mixer. Fix the paddle attachment. Beat the mixture on medium-low speed until creamy.
2. Add in the salt and orange zest. Stir with a wooden spoon.
3. Stir in flour and sugar. Stir until just incorporated. Add nuts and stir. The dough will be dry but it should come together when you press some of it together.
4. Shape the dough into a log of about 2 inches diameter. Wrap the log in cling wrap, waxed paper, or parchment paper and chill for 2–8 hours.
5. Preheat the oven to 350° F. Prepare a baking sheet by lining it with parchment paper.
6. Cut the dough into ¼ inch thick slices. Place the cookies on the baking sheet leaving sufficient gap between them

7. Place the baking sheet in the oven and set the timer for 15–18 minutes or until golden brown around the edges.

8. Let the cookies cool on the baking sheet for about 5–8 minutes. Cool completely on a wire rack.

9. Store in an airtight container. They can up to 10 days in the refrigerator and are delicious from the freezer, where they will keep much longer.

Popped Amaranth

Serves: 3–4

Ingredients:

- 1 cup amaranth seeds

Directions:

1. Place your heaviest pot over medium-high heat. When the pot is nice and hot, add about a tablespoon at a time of amaranth seeds in the pot and spread it evenly. Soon the seeds will start popping. If the pot is not hot, the seeds will not pop and the seeds will have to be discarded.

2. Most seeds will pop. When popping stops, transfer the seeds into a sieve and discard the

seeds that have not popped. Transfer the popped seeds into a bowl.

3. Repeat this process with the remaining seeds. Make sure to pop little seeds at a time.

4. You can season it with salt and pepper and eat it. You can also put it into a bowl of milk and cook it like porridge and eat it. Popped amaranth is also delicious added to other baked recipes such as bars and breads.

Well, now it is time to learn about another category of plant foods that can be foraged in the Mountain West—roots! Read on to learn more!

Chapter 3:

Root It Out

Deep in their roots, all flowers keep the light. –Theodore Roethke

Before looking for edible roots, it's important to understand that there is a difference between roots and tubers. Although people often use these words interchangeably, they are not the same. The root is usually a compact storage organ that has hairy stems developing from the root tissue. Similarly, tubers are also storage organs of the plant, but they don't develop from the root tissue. Instead, tubers develop from the terminal end of stems. So, a plant can have roots as well as tubers. Potatoes are tubers, whereas carrots are roots.

Tubers and roots are incredibly nutritious because the plant's nutrients are stored in these units. When you consume them, the nutrients processed by the plant automatically enter your body. A variety of edible tubers and roots are found in the Mountain West. You will learn about them in this chapter. A wonderful thing about roots and tubers is that they are extremely versatile and can be incorporated into various dishes. They are also packed full of nutrients.

Most root vegetables contain healthy fiber, helpful antioxidants, and low to no cholesterol. As you go through the different root vegetables mentioned in this chapter, you will learn about the different benefits they offer and how to prepare them.

Things to Remember

If you are interested in harvesting roots or tubers, or it is the ideal season to forage for them, carry a trowel or a shovel. Ensure the trowel or shovel you opt for has a comfortable grip and handle and is light. After all, you need to carry it with you wherever you go. This tool ensures that you aren't accidentally damaging the roots or tubers. For instance, haphazardly uprooting a plant because you want its roots might hurt the entire plant, including the edible bits you want to forage. This renders all the efforts made so far useless. Instead, by using a trowel or shovel, you can dig around the plant and slowly dislodge it. The tuber or the roots will be intact when you do this. Also, this method is less invasive and doesn't damage other plants around it. After harvesting the roots or tubers, be sure to cover with soil the trench you dug. After all, any ethical forager aims to not just get what they want from the forest but to leave it in the same or better condition as it was before their interference.

Along with a digging tool, carry sharp shears, and always wear your thick gardening or work gloves (that you have tucked into your sleeves). Handling all the dirt and earth will make your hands dirty and cleaning them in the wild is quite a task. Wearing gloves also reduces the chances of accidentally hurting yourself in this process.

If the root of a specific plant is edible, it's quite likely that other parts of the plant, such as its leaves, stems, and flowers are edible. For instance, this applies to cattails that you will learn about later. You need to be extremely careful while doing this. Don't forget your common sense whenever you are foraging. Also, when it comes to harvesting any edible plant, and especially roots and tubers, ensure they are still young and tender because this is when they taste the best!

The right time to harvest edible roots is fall or early winter. During winter, the ground freezes over in many regions, and digging through the frozen ground isn't possible. This means the roots or tubers will also be hard to access. Also, right before the cold weather sets in, the plants start storing more nutrients in their storage units (roots and tubers) to get through the winter. So, harvesting during autumn or early winter will give you a tasty and sizable harvest!

Common Roots and Tubers to Look For

Now that you know what to carry while looking for roots and tubers in the wild, it is time to learn about common edible varieties found in the Mountain West.

Daylilies

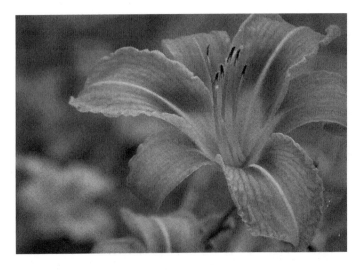

The scientific name of daylily is *Hemerocallis fulva*. The word *Hemerocallis* is derived from two Greek words, *Hemera* and *kallos*, meaning day and beauty, respectively. It was initially native to Asia. However, it was introduced to North America and certain parts of Europe as ornamental plants. These days it can be found along roadsides as well. Even though it's known as a lily, it is nowhere related to the lilies found at the florist, but has similar-looking flowers. The difference is that the flower stalks of the daylily plant are leafless. The primary stem-like leaves are usually up to two feet long and grow directly from the base of the plant instead of the stalk. These plants can be up to four feet tall when mature and grow from thick and fibrous roots.

Different parts of this plant are edible. It's not just the shoots, flower buds, and flowers that are edible. Even the roots can be harvested. While harvesting the shoots, ensure that they are young and tender, and the right time to harvest them is during early spring. This is when the plant is less than eight inches tall. The shoots will be quite tough if the plant is any taller or mature. As soon as the flower stalk is visible, the tubers are depleted and mushy. Therefore, if you want to harvest the tuber, you will need to do it before the flower stalks appear. Therefore, the right time to forage for the tuber is from late fall to early spring.

You don't need any special techniques to use this tuber. Instead, use them just like you would use potatoes. When harvesting the tubers, don't remove the entire clump of roots. Instead, nip one third of it and replant the rest. Doing this will give the plants a chance to regrow, and you will have more to harvest in the future. The flower petals can be dried and added to soups and broths. When fresh, they can be added to salads as well. A word of caution when using daylilies is to always test a sample before eating more because, in some cases, daylilies have been known to cause digestive difficulties and problems.

Cattails

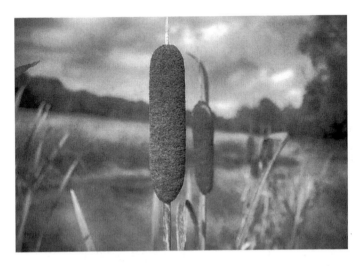

Cattails are commonly found in the wild and are considered to be extremely helpful by survivalists. They belong to the *Typha* genus and include different varieties. The plants are known as cattails because they resemble a cat's tail. You will usually find these plants between early spring and fall. The ideal time to harvest this plant is when it is young and tender. Harvesting as early as possible is suggested because cattails tend to taste quite sweet during this time. Their flavor is often compared to cucumbers and can be eaten in raw and cooked forms.

These plants are native to many regions in both the southern and northern hemispheres and can be found across the Mountain West. Identifying this common plant is easy. Simply look for a plant that resembles a cat's tail. However, the cigar-shaped head isn't formed until the plant fully matures. The young shoots show up in spring, and the plant matures by mid-summer.

Ideally, harvest their shoots and roots when young and tender. Strip away the outer leaves, and you will discover a tender shoot. The tender shoots make a perfect addition to stir-fries. Once dried, cattails can be used to brew herbal teas. Alternatively, freshly harvested cattails can be stored in the freezer for up to three months.

Burdock Root

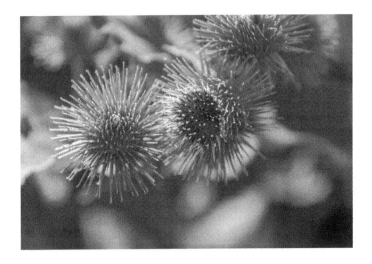

The scientific name of the burdock is *Arctium lappa*. It's also one of the most commonly harvested roots during winter across the Mountain West region. It's quite popular among foragers because its root is believed to have different medicinal properties. Apart from this, it's tasty to consume, and you can harvest this root as long as the ground doesn't freeze during winter. Ideally, the right time to start foraging for burdock root is during the early weeks of winter. As mentioned, it's commonly found across the Mountain West region and almost all over the United States. Florida and Hawaii are the only exceptions.

The simplest way to identify this tree is to look at its leaves. The leaves of the burdock plant are heart shaped. They are white on the underside and green on the outer surface. The leaves can also be up to five to ten centimeters wide when fully mature. Even though these plants can be harvested during winter, doing that is difficult. The roots usually go quite deep in the soil and pulling them out is not easy. As the ground also starts hardening, the job becomes doubly difficult. Ensure you carry a spade or trowel if you wish to harvest burdock or other roots. Dig a trench around the plant to harvest burdock root and slowly scoop it out.

Burdock root can be used in fresh and dried forms. Once fully dry, it can be powdered and added to any other recipe. When fresh, it can be eaten raw, sauteed, or stir-fried.

Kudzu

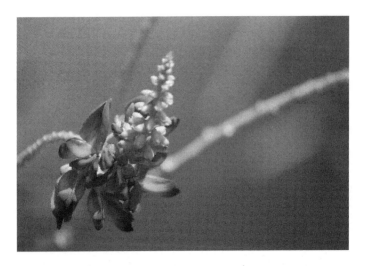

The scientific name of kudzu is *Pueraria montana.* This twining vine is a perennial and belongs to the Fabaceae or pea family. Though native to Asia, it was introduced sometime during the 1800s to the US to regulate soil erosion and for livestock to forage. It grows quite quickly and can grow up to 30 cm on a given day; therefore, it is also known as the mile-a-minute vine. These vines easily coil and climb anything that comes their way. You will commonly find them in open fields, edges of forests, fields, and roadsides. Kudzu is a hardy plant and does well in all types of soil, especially deep and well-drained loamy soil. It also prefers sunny areas and, in addition to the Mountain West, it is commonly found in the southern, central, and eastern US and in the Pacific Northwest.

When fully mature, these plants can be up to 10-30 meters long. Since it is a vine, you cannot measure its height; instead, its length is measured. This yellow-green vine can be up to 10 inches wide in some cases. It has long and bristly leaves that can be up to six inches each. It produces red-purple flowers with a yellow spot on the flower's stem. The blossoms usually appear between June and September. The compound and alternate leaves have three leaflets.

The leaves, vine tips, roots, and flowers are all edible. The fragrant flowers are commonly added to jellies, syrups, and candies. The root can be cooked just like potatoes. The starch extracted from it is commonly used as a batter for deep-fried foods. It can also be used as a thickener.

Recipes

Here are some delicious recipes incorporating the nutritious roots and tubers you gathered in the Mountain West region. Don't hesitate to experiment with the ingredients once you get the hang of how to prepare them and the flavor combination.

Daylily Flower Fritters

Serves: 3–4

Ingredients:

- 10–15 daylily flowers and large almost open buds
- ½ cup milk
- ½ teaspoon baking powder
- vegetable oil to fry, as required
- ½ cup flour + extra to dredge
- ¼ teaspoon salt
- spices of your choice
- water, as required

Directions:

1. Combine flour, baking powder, salt, spices, and milk in a bowl. Stir until smooth and free from lumps.
2. Add a little water if the batter is very thick or if the batter is runny, add more flour.
3. Add some flour into a shallow bowl.
4. Pour about 2 inches of oil in a heavy bottomed pan. Place the pan over medium-high heat. Wait until the oil is hot but not smoking, around 365° F.
5. Roll the buds and flowers in flour. Shake off extra flour and dip in the batter one at a time and gently slide it into the hot oil.
6. Add as many as can fit in the pan. Cook the remaining in batches. Cook until the fritters are golden brown. Turn occasionally.

7. Remove the fritters with a slotted spoon and place on a plate lined with paper towels.
8. Serve hot with a dip of your choice.

Cattail Stalk Hot Dill Pickles

Serves: 15 - 20

Ingredients:

- 12–15 young cattail stalk shoots, cleaned, discard outer layers
- ½ bunch dill
- 4 cloves garlic, peeled
- 3 bay leaves
- 3 dried chili peppers or 3 slivers fresh habanero pepper (optional)

For brine:

- 2 ½ cups water
- 3 ½ tablespoons kosher salt
- 2 ½ cups white vinegar

Directions:

1. Dry the cattail stalk shoots by patting with a kitchen towel. Cut them into about 4 inch pieces. Place the stalks in sterilized jars. Stuff

the garlic and chili peppers in between the stalks, at different places.

2. To make brine: Mix together water, salt, and vinegar into a saucepan. Place the saucepan over medium high heat. When it starts boiling, turn off the heat.
3. Pour the brine into the jar, all over the cattail stalks.
4. Meanwhile, set up a water bath for canning the pickle. Follow the manufacturer's instructions on the procedure.
5. Place the jar in the water bath for 5 minutes.
6. Label the jar with name and date.
7. Store in a cool and dark area.
8. In case you do not want to place the jars in the water bath, place the jars in the refrigerator. They can last a few weeks in the refrigerator.

Roasted Burdock Roots

Serves: 3–4

Ingredients:

- 1 pound burdock roots, cut into 1 inch round slices
- ½ teaspoon salt or to taste
- 1 tablespoon extra-virgin olive oil
- ½ teaspoon pepper

- Sesame seeds
- soy sauce

Directions:

1. Preheat the oven to 400° F.
2. Put burdock root slices in a bowl. Add oil, pepper, and salt. Mix well.
3. Transfer the burdock slices onto a baking sheet and spread the slices in a single layer.
4. Place the baking sheet in the oven and set the timer for about 15 to 17 minutes. Flip sides and continue baking until golden brown on the outside and cooked through inside.

Kudzu Tea (Arrowroot Tea)

Serves: 2

Ingredients:

- 2 tablespoons kudzu root powder
- 2 cups cold water
- honey or brown sugar to taste

Optional ingredients:

- ¼ teaspoon ground ginger
- ¼ teaspoon ground cinnamon

- ½ teaspoon matcha tea powder

Directions:

1. Add kudzu powder, water, sweetener, and any one or all of the optional ingredients into a saucepan. Stir until well combined.
2. Place the saucepan over medium-low heat. Stir constantly until the mixture becomes clear (semi-transparent). Turn off the heat and cool for a few minutes. This is to be served warm.
3. Pour into cups and serve.

Various foods found in the Mountain West region cannot be confined to a single category. Therefore, you need to learn more! The next step toward becoming a forager is learning about different edible greens that can be foraged.

Chapter 4:

Fields of Green

Salad can get a bad rap. People think of bland and watery iceberg lettuce, but salads are an art form, from the simplest rendition to a colorful kitchen-sink approach. –Marcus Samuelsson

Greens harvested from the wild are filled with a variety of healthy antioxidants and nutrients. Incorporating leafy greens into your diet is one of the best means to improve your health. They are packed full of vitamins and minerals. Combining these factors can improve your overall health and provide your body with the nutrition it needs.

Eating greens is not new, and humans have been doing it since prehistoric times. Dark green leafy vegetables, salad greens, or any other green leafy vegetables are usually rich in vitamins A and K. They also contain carotenoids. These antioxidants tackle the damage caused by oxidative stress and inflammation. They also have high fiber, magnesium, calcium, and potassium levels. Whether you want to add the greens to a salad or soup or turn it into a smoothie, go ahead and do it. Try to ensure that you eat green leafy vegetables, in some form or another, daily.

Things to Remember

Whenever you harvest greens, it is best to do it early in the day. This is because the greens usually taste better before the sun hits them. Similarly, always opt for young and tender greens because they taste the best. As the plant matures, its foliage also toughens up and can become quite bitter in most cases. In some cases, the mature varieties can even become inedible, and the body cannot digest it. The best way to harvest them is to carry a pair of sharp scissors or garden shears, and remember to wear gloves. This is especially needed whenever you are handling plants in the wild. While foraging, the chances of accidentally touching any prickly plants or coming into contact with any toxic substances produced by poisonous plants reduces when you wear gloves.

If you are interested in harvesting greens, you must also carry a basket. Regardless of how sturdy or comfortable a backpack is, you will also need a basket. Greens and other plant foliage are delicate and, if not handled properly, will be squished and lose their shape and texture. You will need something to carry them to ensure this does not happen. This is where a basket steps into the picture. Also, carry paper bags for different plant foods you forage and label them. This makes it easier to identify or separate the greens later. When it comes to foraging, as with any other activity in life, a little planning and preparation go a long way in making the entire job more comfortable and convenient.

When it comes to greens, many poisonous look-alikes exist, and you need to be aware of them. Ensure that you do not eat or even handle a plant when in doubt. If you are unsure, stay away from the plant; you can always get back to it later. You could draw it or take a photo and ask local experts once you get back home.

Another important thing you must remember while harvesting greens is not to destroy the entire plant. If you know that you will only use a specific plant's tender stems or leaves, what is the point of uprooting it? Be respectful and mindful of nature. You must become an ethical forager and not destroy anything by pillaging. Also, do not harvest more than one-third of the plant and one-third of the given patch at any point. This practice ensures the plants can thrive and regrow.

Common Greens to Look For

You will come across a variety of edible greens while foraging in the Mountain West region. However, don't harvest anything before properly identifying it. Remember the above-mentioned considerations and read on to discover common edible greens!

Sumac

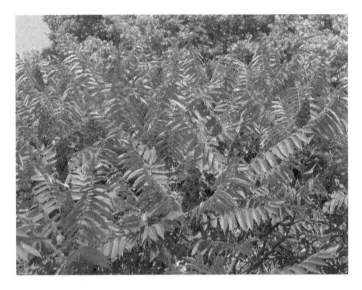

The scientific name of staghorn sumac is *Rhus typhina*, and it is a deciduous shrub native to the United States and Canada. You'll find plenty of it, especially from mid to late summer. Here is a fun fact about this plant—it belongs to the cashew family! Whenever you are foraging for staghorn sumac, be mindful of poison sumac. Even though the poisonous leaves are somewhat similar to the edible variety, poison sumac is incredibly harmful to humans. The primary difference you need to remember is that poison sumac has clusters of white-gray berries that hang downwards and grow exclusively in damp or flooded areas such as swamps. As a rule of thumb, avoid all plants that have white berries! So, if a plant looks like sumac but has white berries, then chances are it is poisonous.

Edible staghorn sumac has alternate compound leaves that can be up to 60 cm long when fully mature. Its rounded and narrow leaflets have a pointy tip and serrated edges. The leaflets themselves are smooth and dark green on the outer surface, whereas pale on the undersurface. Edible sumac features clusters of greenish-yellow flowers from June until July. Each flower has five petals and looks quite pretty. This particular variety of sumac gets its name from the velvety young branches resembling a young stag's antlers. The immature or young growing branches are usually brown and smooth. During winter, you might notice U-shaped leaf scars on it. When it grows outdoors, it can be up to seven meters tall. The trunk itself can be up to four feet wide or more. It is usually dark brown and smooth, but the older barks are grayish-brown.

Between August and September, this plant sports fruits. The fruiting head consists of a cluster of compact, round, and red hairy fruits known as drupes. Each drupe has one seed, and each cluster can contain anywhere between 100 to 700 seeds. Until the tree is three to four years old, it doesn't start fruiting. It is not just the edible fruits; even the young shoots can be consumed. The shoots need to be peeled and then eaten. However, it is too old to be palatable if you see a pith or an off-white core inside the shoot. The shoots must be green on the inside. If they are, simply remove the outer covering, and cook them like any other greens.

Sassafras

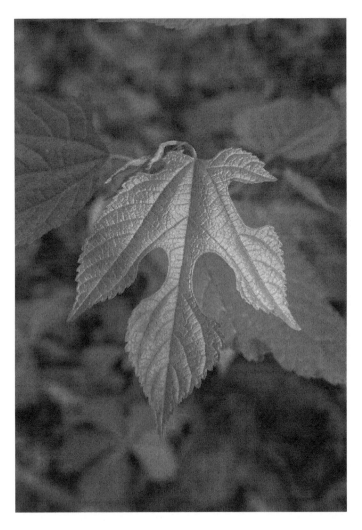

The scientific name of sassafras is *Sassafras albidum*. This tree is native to North America, and its roots and bark were commonly used to make herbal tea. Its dried and powdered leaves are often used in cooking gumbo and are known as Filé. A word of caution about sassafras is that their roots and bark contain a chemical known as safrole. Safrole was declared a carcinogen by the US Food and Drug Administration during the 1960s. However, if they are consumed in small doses as indigenous peoples usually do, sassafras roots and bark can possibly be considered safe. The leaves don't contain this compound, so they are considered safe for human consumption. This deciduous tree can be up to 20 meters tall when fully mature and has a deeply fissured dark reddish-brown bark. Its lobed leaves are its characteristic feature. The leaves resemble a mitten with one or two thumbs on either side. You might even come across sassafras leaves with more than three lobes. During fall, the leaves take on a yellowish orange hue and are a sight to behold.

These plants are found across many parts of the United States, including the Mountain West. Depending on what you intend to use sassafras for, the foraging seasons differ. If you want green leaves, then you must forage them from early spring until fall. If you want the roots or the bark, you can harvest anytime. The leaves can be used to flavor soups and sauces. As I mentioned, sassafras is commonly used as a thickener in Creole cooking when dried and powdered. The leaves can also be steeped in hot water to brew herbal tea. Until the 1960s, sassafras used to be the star ingredient in the soft drinks "sarsaparilla" and some "root beer," until safety concerns arose.

Field garlic

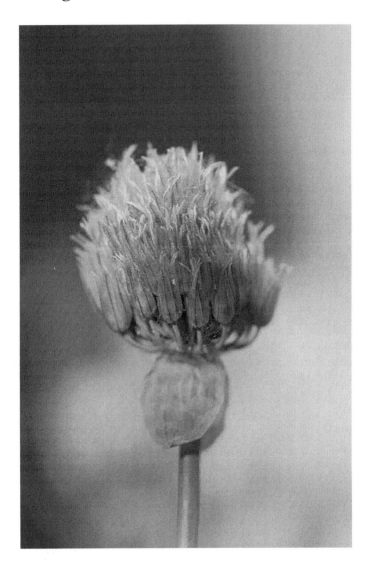

The scientific name of field garlic is *Allium vineale*. It is pretty much found everywhere across the United States. You can count on foraging wild garlic even during the cold winter months. It's also commonly referred to as wild chives, wild garlic, and onion grass. This is one of those plants that is not only hardy but is found almost everywhere. These plants are ephemeral, meaning when the soil starts to heat up as summer approaches, the plant dies. However, as the weather cools down, the plant reappears. So, this plant is self-seeding.

You need to be extra careful when identifying field garlic because it has look-alikes. Some look-alikes are harmless, such as chives, but others are poisonous. For instance, field garlic's slim, narrow, tubular, and hollow leaves resemble wild onions. On the other hand, another look-alike of these plants is fly poison. These plants look like field garlic, including their tubular stem structure and flowers, but are harmful to humans. Another species you must watch out for is the death camas. So, learning to identify field garlic properly is the best way to ensure that you don't unknowingly eat any other poisonous plant.

Field garlic usually has slender and tubular green leaves that are hollow on the inside. The leaves can be up to two feet tall, and the entire plant has a strong onion-like smell. The bulb of this plant must look like miniature onions growing together in small clusters. When this plant blooms during late spring, the flowers are pink or white colored. Ensure that the plant you are looking at satisfies all the conditions mentioned above, and once you have consulted experts as needed and are completely sure, only then should you go ahead and harvest.

Usually, you will find these plants in open woods and fields across the United States. Winter and fall are the right time to harvest them. Assuming you correctly identified it, the entire plant is edible and can be harvested. However, ensure that you avoid harvesting all of the field garlic from the same spot. If a portion of it is harvested, it will regrow. However, if you uproot an entire patch without leaving behind even a single plant, it cannot regrow. So, as an ethical forager, only harvest one-third of any patch whenever you come across field garlic. Make a note of the spot and revisit over time.

Avoid foraging any plants from any visibly polluted areas, and this is especially important when it comes to field garlic. Any toxins, heavy metals, or chemicals found in the soil are automatically absorbed by most plants, and especially by this one.

The pungent onion-like tasting plant comes with a hint of garlic flavor. Any recipe that utilizes chives or onions will do well with field garlic. The green tops can be used just like chives, whereas bulbs can be used as a replacement for onions.

Dooryard Violet

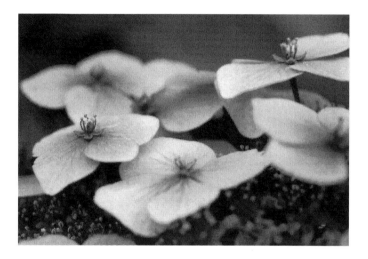

The scientific name of dooryard violet is *Viola sororia*. Violets bloom in abundance from early spring until mid-summer. Leaves, as well as flowers of this plant, are edible. Even though most only think of violets as purely ornamental plants, they have different culinary applications too. These plants usually prefer cooler climates but not extreme cold. In regions where the winters are relatively warm, violets can also be harvested later in the year. They are native to the rocky parts of the US, especially in the Mountain West region. If you are native to the United States, chances are you know how violets look. That said, learning to properly identify them is important to ensure you don't confuse them with their poisonous look-alikes. The simplest way to identify this plant is to look at its leaves. The heart-shaped leaves have a pointed tip with rounded teeth-like margins along the edges.

The simplest way to harvest it is by pulling up the plant. Do this only if you will use its stems and roots, and don't over-harvest in the area. You will usually find violets along roadsides and other open areas. That said, avoid harvesting anything from busy, polluted highway roadsides. Use your problem-solving and common sense to avoid problems. The leaves and flowers can alternatively be plucked depending on your needs. The leaves and flowers are rich in vitamins A and C. The flowers can be used as an edible garnish or candied too. The leaves can be added to salads when young and tender. You can also dry these parts of this plant and use them to brew herbal teas.

Plantain

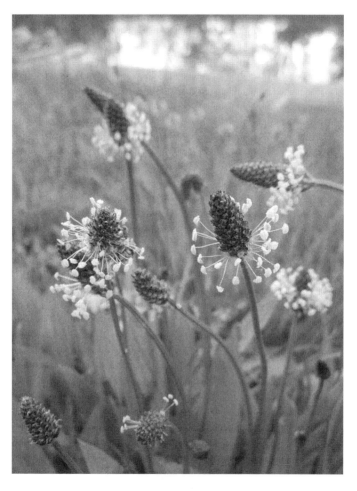

The scientific name of plantain is *Plantago Ianceolata*. This is a medicinal plant that usually shows up from spring until the end of summer. There are two varieties of this plant, narrow leaf plantain and broadleaf plantain. The broadleaf plantain is commonly found across the United States and is widely foraged. It is native to most parts of Northern and Central Asia and Europe; however, this plant has also spread to different parts of the world. They usually grow on lawns, along busy roadsides, and in other areas experiencing human activity. It prefers well-distributed and compact soil.

You can identify the broadleaf plantain with its oval and egg-shaped green leaves. The leaves usually grow in a rosette, with heavy stems covering the entire base of the plant. When young, this green plant doesn't have any stems per se. The leaves are a particular delicacy and are also used as a vegetable. While harvesting the leaves, the right time is to pick them early in the day or after the sun goes down. Harvest these leaves as you would have harvested spinach or kale. Ensure that you are quite careful while harvesting them and stay away from infected or unhealthy leaves.

You can either consume the fresh leaves raw or in cooked forms. Ideally, opt for young leaves because they taste the best. When placed in the refrigerator, these leaves will stay fresh for up to a week. By the way, this plant's small, edible seeds are often found in health food stores labeled "psyllium husks."

Pokeweed

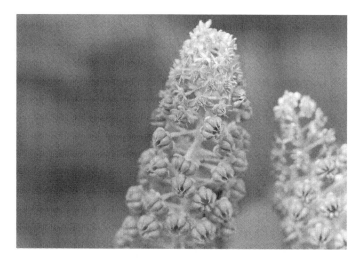

Phytolacca americana is the scientific name of pokeweed. Even though its greens can be considered edible, they must not be eaten raw. Also, avoid touching any part of this plant with your bare hands because the toxins secreted by it cause skin irritation and other harmful and often painful symptoms. This is because the skin easily absorbs the toxins secreted by it. If you eat any part of this plant in its raw form, including its roots, common symptoms associated with pokeweed poisoning can develop, such as convulsions, vomiting, and respiratory distress.

This herbaceous perennial plant grows into a large bush that can be up to 10 feet tall when fully mature. Due to its height, it is commonly mistaken for a tree instead of a bush. This plant has purple and red stems along with an extensive taproot system. The hairless and smooth-to-touch stems have oval-shaped leaves. The leaves are quite long, and during the early weeks of autumn, you'll notice purple berries on this plant. Even though these berries resemble small grapes, avoid eating them because they are harmful to humans.

Watercress

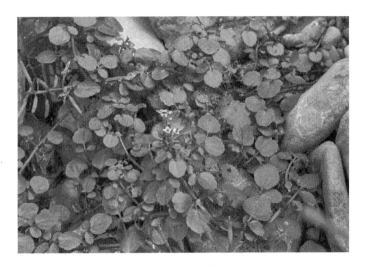

An interesting fact about the leaves of the watercress plant is that they will stay green throughout winter. The scientific name of the watercress is *Nasturtium officinale*. These peppery and punchy greens are commonly used in salads and are quite popular with foragers because they are fairly easy to identify and are found in most regions. This plant is believed to be native to Europe and the United States. These delicious leaves have been harvested for culinary purposes for ages. The common areas where watercress is found within the United States include the cold alkaline waters of springs and other water bodies. It's commonly prevalent in the western part of the United States but has spread toward the north as well.

This glossy-looking plant is medium-sized and has smooth leaves. It's usually found in aquatic as well as subaquatic regions. The easiest way to identify it is by paying attention to its flowers. This plant sports clusters of small white flowers during summer, but it can also be harvested in winter. If you want to harvest watercress plants, you simply need to cut the leaves and a little bit of the stem with it. Harvest the leaves and stems a couple of inches above the ground using a sharp knife or a pair of scissors. Ensure that you do not pull or roughly tug the stem. Instead, leave its roots as undisturbed as possible to ensure that it keeps growing.

If you want to enjoy watercress, ensure that you consume it immediately after harvest. You can add them to a salad or consume in cooked forms too. Refrigerating or freezing the leaves prolongs its shelf-life.

Dandelions

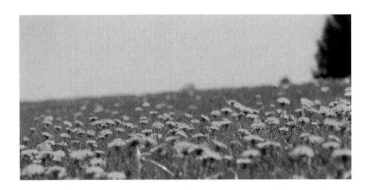

Dandelions are one of the most popular flowers worldwide, and their scientific name is *Taraxacum officinale*. They're not only known for their pretty yellow flowers but have different medicinal as well as culinary applications too. Almost every part of this plant is edible, including its roots, flowers, and leaves. They are also fairly easy to identify and can be ideal for foragers of all levels of experience.

This plant is found across all regions of North America and is usually found in abandoned fields and roadsides (and many back yards). The plants bloom during early spring and are fully mature by mid-summer. The simplest way to identify this plant is to look for its yellow flowers and basal leaves. The leaves grow from the bottom of the stem, and the flower grows on a single unbranching stem that is hollow. The stem, along with the lobed leaves, usually produces a milky white sap when cut. The flower head is around two inches wide and consists of hundreds of ray-shaped flowers produced in clusters. This plant's hollow stem can be between two and 24 inches tall.

Since the entire plant is edible, you can harvest whatever is needed. For instance, if you only want to harvest the greens, snap or cut the leaves or the young stems. The leaves are tender in spring and fall and are best picked in the early morning. Ensure you do not uproot the entire plant if you don't want to use the entire plant.

Ideally, harvest the leaves right before the plant blooms because they taste best when tender. Also, as the plants mature, the leaves take on a slightly bitter taste. The flavor profile of dandelion greens is quite similar to that of arugula. The leaves can be added to salads and stir-fries. You can also dry the leaves and flowers and brew herbal tea with them.

Recipes

Whether it is field garlic, watercress, or some other lovely green edible plant, if you have managed to get your hands on these delicious and nutritious ingredients, it is time to start using them! This section will cover extremely simple recipes that honor the ingredients foraged in the Mountain West!

Plantain Weed Salad

Serves: 7–8

Ingredients:

- 4 cups finely chopped plantain leaf weeds
- 2 cans (28 ounces each) chickpeas, drained, rinsed
- 2 stalks celery, finely chopped
- 1 cup finely chopped cabbage
- 2 onions, chopped
- 3–4 cloves garlic, peeled, finely chopped
- ¼ cup wine vinegar
- ¼ cup olive oil
- salt to taste

Directions:

1. Add plantain weeds, chickpeas, celery, cabbage, onion, and garlic into a bowl and toss well.
2. Cover the bowl and chill until use.
3. Just before serving, pour vinegar and oil over the salad. Toss well.
4. Season with salt and serve.

Wild Garlic Pesto

Serves: 15–20

Ingredients:

- 2 large bunches wild garlic, washed well
- 4.2 ounces pine nuts, toasted
- 10 ounces olive oil
- salt to taste
- 2 small bunches curly parsley, washed well
- 4.2 ounces parmesan cheese
- 1 tablespoon lemon juice or to taste
- pepper to taste

Directions:

1. Place wild garlic, pine nuts, salt, parsley, parmesan, lemon juice, and pepper in a blender and blend until smooth.
2. With the blender machine running, pour oil in a thin drizzle. Blend until well combined.
3. Pour into a bowl. Chill until use. You can use it for pastas, pizzas, as a spread, etc.

Gingered Watercress

Serves: 3

Ingredients:

- 12 ounces fresh watercress, trimmed, rinsed, spin dried
- 1 clove garlic, minced

- ¼ cup chopped tomatoes
- 1 inch fresh ginger, peeled, minced
- freshly ground pepper to taste
- salt to taste

Directions:

1. Pour oil into a skillet and let it heat over medium-high heat. When the oil is hot, add ginger and garlic and cook for a few seconds until you get a nice aroma. Make sure not to burn it.
2. Stir in tomatoes and cook until soft. Stir in the watercress and cook until tender and they wilt.
3. Add salt and pepper to taste and serve.

Dandelion Pizza

Serves: 8

Ingredients:

- 2 cups dandelion flowers and greens
- 4 tablespoons butter
- 1 teaspoon minced basil
- 1 teaspoon minced, fresh rosemary
- 2 tablespoons minced garlic
- ½ cup heavy cream
- salt to taste
- 2 cups pizza sauce

- 8 flatbreads or 2 prebaked pizza crusts
- 4 cups shredded mozzarella cheese

Directions:

1. Add butter into a skillet and let it melt over medium heat. When butter melts, add dandelion flowers and greens and stir fry for 1–2 minutes.
2. Stir in garlic, herbs, cream, and salt. Cook until nearly dry.
3. Preheat the oven to 425° F.
4. Place flatbreads on a large baking sheet and put it into the oven.
5. Bake for about 4 minutes.
6. Remove the baking sheet from the oven. Divide the pizza sauce equally and spread it over the flatbreads.
7. Divide the cooked dandelion leaves on top of the flatbreads. Scatter cheese on top.
8. Bake until the cheese is brown at a few spots.
9. Serve hot.

Well, are you eager to learn more about other foods that can be foraged? Now, let's get to the juicy bit, pun intended! It is time to learn about the berries as well as fruits that can be foraged.

Chapter 5:

Juicy Goodness

Summer in Seattle allows me to indulge in some of the region's top culinary delights - I'm talking about wild king salmon and fresh, ripe Washington stone fruits and berries like cherries, peaches, plums, and blueberries. –Tom Douglas

Have you ever walked by a bush of berries and wondered if they were edible? Or perhaps you have seen delicious looking fruit but didn't know if you could eat them? Well, with some information and the right knowledge, you can quickly identify different varieties of berries and fruits in the wild. Different types of edible berries gathered in the wild are filled with nature's goodness, and you can obtain the benefits they offer by simply adding them to your diet.

Regardless of whether they are blueberries, wild strawberries, or common chokeberry and persimmons, there are different varieties that you can forage in the wild. Each of them offers a variety of nutrients and has interesting flavor profiles. From jams and jellies to pies and other desserts, fruits and berries can be easily incorporated into daily meals. All it requires is a little conscious decision-making. So, why should you add these ingredients to your diet?

Berries are among the healthiest foods you can eat. They are loaded with helpful antioxidants known to regulate oxidative stress and reduce the risk of cellular degeneration. Regular consumption of berries and other fruits also improves the antioxidant level in the body, which in turn is good for improving the health of your skin. Regular consumption of berries is known to stabilize blood sugar levels and offer the body the required fiber. Most of the carbohydrates present in them are in the form of fiber, which is desirable. So, you can eat plenty of berries without worrying about raising your sugar level.

Things to Remember

You must carry a basket whenever you want to harvest fruits or berries! They are delicate, especially when ripe, and can get squished easily. If the fruit is squished, then there isn't much you can do about it later. Usually, the best way to go about harvesting fruits or berries, especially the ripe ones, is to place a blanket or a tarp under the tree and then shake the tree. If it is a bush, then you can simply pluck the fruit you need. Once again, don't harvest more than $1/3^{rd}$ of the berries or fruit you come across. Other foragers, as well as local wildlife, will also want to eat it. And remember, don't damage the entire plant if all you want are its berries or fruits.

Avoid eating any berries directly off the plant in the wild unless you are 100% certain of their identity. The berries may look delicious and tempting, but that doesn't mean they are edible. Likewise, just because they look like something familiar doesn't make them edible. So, take photos and ask experts after your first few trips. Once you are completely certain, then you might start picking. And as one (of many) important rules of thumb, avoid all plants that have white berries!

Berries and Fruits to Look For

Foraging for berries and fruits is quite exciting. These ingredients are not only versatile but can be incorporated into different dishes as well. From jams and preserves to salads, smoothies, and pies, you can use them in a variety of preparations. Here are some common edible berries and fruits you will find in the Mountain West region.

Wild Strawberry

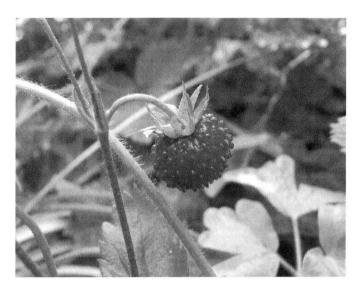

Strawberries can also easily forage in the wild, and they are scientifically known as *Fragaria virginiana*. Wild strawberry is a herbaceous perennial plant native to North America and can be found in the Mountain West region. Identifying this plant is especially easy due to its characteristic leaves with serrated edges and fuzzy undersides covered with fine hair-like structures. The five-petaled white flowers of this plant have a yellow center and bloom in clusters between April and June. The long and hairy runners of this plant usually reroot and result in the growth of new plantlets. Toward the end of the blooming season, the flowers are replaced by small and rounded red strawberries! The leaves are bright green on the upper surface and slightly paler on the underside.

The flowers, leaves, and fruits are this plant's edible parts. It is also known as scarlet strawberry due to its bright red color. Apart from this, the strawberries found in the wild are tastier than the commercially cultivated ones. This plant's young and tender leaves can be used to brew herbal teas or added to salads. Once you get your hands on some wild strawberries, you have different options available to prepare or cook them. When you are completely sure what you have found, the most obvious option is to eat the red and luscious berries right off the plant! You can add them to salads, turn them into jam, jelly, or syrup, or even incorporate them into any dessert of your choice! It can be added to juices and smoothies as well. The options are truly endless when it comes to preparing this delicious fruit.

Wild Black Cherry

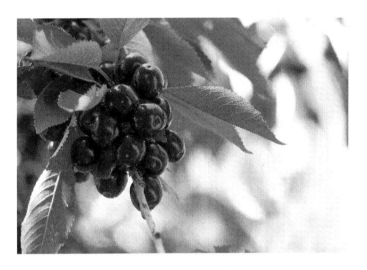

The scientific name of the black cherry is *Prunus avium*. If you are foraging during summer, keep an eye out for these delicious berries. These wild cherries are quite similar in taste to commercially cultivated cherries. They are also known as the better cousin of chokecherries because of their similar appearance. These trees are commonly found along the Eastern coast of the US, Central US, and into eastern Texas. So, you will find them in the Mountain West region quite easily, provided you know what you are looking for.

Unlike blueberries and strawberries that grow on bushes, black cherries grow on tall and straight trees with shaggy and thick trunks. These beautiful trees usually form a canopy in forests, and harvesting the berries is not an easy task. As the tree matures, the lenticular stripes on the bark slowly develop, and take on their characteristic shaggy appearance. The long, narrow, and dark green leaves have slightly serrated margins and a central vein. The leaves resemble that of chokecherry, as well as regular cherry trees. It doesn't start blooming until the tree is around 15 feet tall. When it blooms, you will notice flower spikes.

The slightly red berries take on a deep shade as they mature and almost look black. Though these berries are small, they are extremely delicious and filled with various helpful nutrients. Adding these wild berries to your diet can work wonders for your health, because they contain vitamin C and antioxidants. The cherries are perfectly ripe as soon as they come off the stem when you touch them. Alternatively, pick only the dark berries if you want to eat them immediately. If you are plucking the unripe berries, give them a few days to ripen and then eat. They can be eaten raw or added to jams, jellies, and syrups. Use them like you would use regular cherries.

Avoid eating the black cherry pits because, upon consumption, a compound present in them is actively converted into hydrocyanic acid. This is quite harmful to humans. However, the flesh is considered safe to eat!

Blueberries

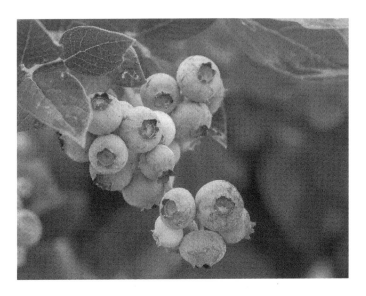

Blueberries are among the most popular berries consumed across the world. The blue and round berries are incredibly juicy and tasty and offer a variety of nutritional values, too. The scientific name of blueberries is *Vaccinium sect. Cyanococcus*. This perennial flower plant produces juicy blue or purple berries and belongs to the *Vaccinium* genus. This genus also houses other popular berries such as cranberries, bilberries, and huckleberries. While foraging for blueberries, look for other plants with similar berries because they all belong to the same family. However, ensure that you have correctly identified the berries before eating them. As a rule, stay away from any plant with white berries.

Blueberries are commonly found across the Mountain West region. The varieties of blueberries found in the wild are the same as the ones cultivated commercially across the globe. A significant portion of blueberries produced within the United States are obtained from the regions of Washington, Oregon, Michigan, California, North Carolina, Texas, New Jersey, and Minnesota. These berries grow freely in most areas, and you will find them along roadsides, in forests, and abandoned fields. You will also come across them in National Forests, as well as parks. Before you start foraging in a National Park or forest, ensure that you have read through the legal requirements and have the needed permits in place.

Any species of blueberry that grows within the United States produces round fruits in shades of blue or dark purple. The distinctive characteristic of this fruit is its 5-pointed crown that's immediately visible. The thin branches producing light pink or white colored flowers are another identifying factor of this plant. The leaves of this plant are usually dark green with hints of yellow. The leaves are smooth and grow in clusters of six or fewer. The leaves are oval or egg-shaped and wider at the bottom than the top.

Blueberries are rich in various nutrients and filled with antioxidants. Regular consumption of blueberries reduces cholesterol, tackles high blood pressure, and reduces the risk of cardiovascular diseases. The antioxidants in them are also known to fight inflammation. Harvesting blueberries is incredibly simple. You simply need to pluck the fruit or use a special rake brush to collect the berries. Don't forget to carry a basket to keep the foraged berries intact. Once the berries take on a dark blue color and are slightly soft to the touch, they are perfectly ripe and ready for consumption. You can eat them directly or add them to various dishes, such as pies or cakes. Blueberries can also be turned into jams or jellies.

Juneberries

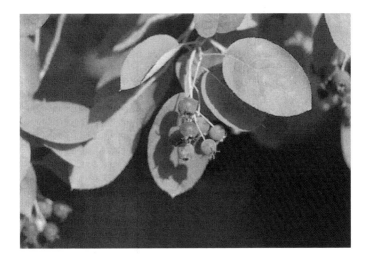

The scientific name of Juneberry is *Amelanchier laevis* and is commonly known as serviceberry. When the berries are fully ripe, they resemble blueberries. The juicy and delicious berries are filled with different nutrients, including the body's vitamin C and antioxidants. Juneberries are commonly found in open woodlands, lakesides, and city parks. They thrive in full sunlight and are usually tall shrubs. These plants are native to North America.

Even though the berries resemble blueberries when fully mature, juneberries are closer to apples and pears than other berries. They resemble blueberries because of their five-pointed crown associated with a typical blueberry. The berries are usually green to begin with, and then take on a deep red color. When fully ripe, they resemble purple more than red. The flowers of this plant usually bloom before any of the leaves emerge. The five-petalled white flowers are a key part of identifying this plant. The leaves themselves are oval-shaped and unfurl alternatively on the stalks. The leaves have serrated margins. The foliage takes on a golden-amber shade during autumn. The gray bark of this plant usually develops shallow grooves as it matures. Harvesting these berries is incredibly easy. Berries are the only edible part of this plant. Usually, you will find ripe juneberries from late spring until early summer. Once harvested, you can use them just like any other berries. You can add them to pies and other desserts, along with jams and jellies. The berries can be frozen and stored for later too. These mild and sweet berries are truly a delight to forage.

Persimmons

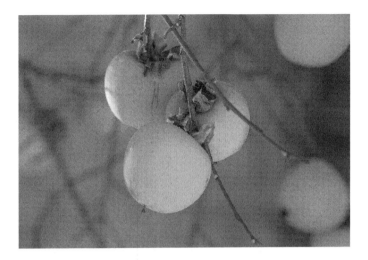

One of the easily recognizable fruits in the wild is the American Persimmon, scientifically known as *Diospyros kaki*. It's also a popular cultivated plant, and is usually available in most supermarkets and grocery stores. Asian persimmon is the cultivated variety, whereas the persimmons found in the wild are much smaller and similar to cherry tomatoes in size. These are commonly found in the Mountain West region and eastern hardwood forests within the United States. These fruits are rich in vitamins A and C and are pulpy and sweet. They also have a hint of spiciness. Usually, these fruits ripen during November. Harvested before the fruit fully matures, it will be slightly bitter. The red or yellow fruits are around 2-3-inches wide.

A simple way to identify this plant is to look at its bark. The dark bark has visible patterns of blocks along with vertical ridges running along the length of its trunk. The thin and smooth twigs and branches of this tree are grayish-brown. The fruits usually form in small clusters and are incredibly juicy. When you bite into it, you'll notice flattened seeds. The oval or elliptic-oblong-shaped leaves are 2.5 to 6 cm long and grow alternatively on the branches. The upper surface of the leaf is medium to dark green and glossy, whereas its lower pale green surface is leathery and soft to the touch. The fruits can also be eaten fresh, stewed, or turned into a jam.

Red Mulberry

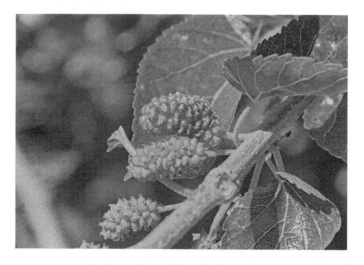

The red mulberry was initially native to the regions of Asia and, in particular, China. It was introduced in northern America during the 1600s and started gaining popularity thereon. These trees played a vital role in silk production because their leaves are the preferred food for silkworms. Silk is extracted from these worms. The scientific name of this tree is *Morbus alba*.

The delicious berries produced by this tree are commonly found toward the end of May and stay on for a couple of months after that. The oval and cylindrical fruits are initially greenish or white, to begin with, and take on their typical reddish-purple color as they mature. As soon as the berries are dark and slightly soft to the touch, they're fully ripe and fit for consumption. This tree is characterized by its short white trunks and thin bark that goes from light brown to gray as it starts maturing. The leaves are found in an alternative pattern on their stems. The broad leaves have three prominent veins that are evident upon inspection. These leaves are a shiny green color on the outer surface and pale on the underside. These plants usually flower between April and May, depending on the geographical location. You will find these delicious berries across the Mountain West region. The berries are filled with a variety of vitamins and antioxidants. They can be eaten fresh or even stored for later. They can be added to salads, syrups, jams, and jellies. When frozen, they last for a couple of months if stored properly.

Red Chokecherry

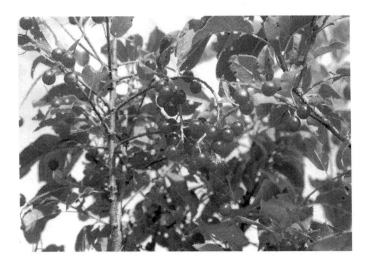

Chokecherries are commonly confused with black cherries because they all belong to the same genus, *Prunus*. The scientific name of these berries is *Prunus virginiana*. Even though some categorize it as a tree, it's actually a shrub belonging to the rose family. These plants can be over 20 feet tall when fully mature and are, therefore, known as trees. Chokecherries are also known as red cherries or eastern chokecherries. They are commonly found across the United States, especially in rocky areas. So, if you are living in (or visiting) the Mountain West, you very well may find red chokecherries in the wild.

The simplest way to identify red chokecherry is to look at its leaves that grow alternatively on the stem. The long leaves are oval-shaped with a hairy tip and serrated edges. Toward the upper part of the tree, its leaves are usually darker than the ones closer to the base. Between May and June, flowers bloom on this plant in cylindrical clusters. During late summer, purple or red colored fruit starts appearing. Their light brown or gray stems are slender. Break a twig, and you will notice an unpleasant odor. If you don't notice the smell, you have wrongly identified the plant.

If you are absolutely certain of what they are, the red berries can be eaten right off the tree when fully ripe. You can also consume them in cooked forms. Do not eat the pit of this fruit because it contains hydrocyanic acid that's poisonous to humans. The fruit flesh is the only edible part of this plant and avoid eating any other part.

Recipes

Well, after reading about the different edible berries and fruits that can be foraged in the wild, you may be excited to get started. Here are some incredibly simple and mouth-watering recipes that will help make the most of the ingredients foraged.

Wild Strawberry Jam

Makes: 2 jars

Ingredients:

- 3 cups wild strawberries, discard stems
- 1 ½ cups sugar
- ½ teaspoon Pomona's pectin powder
- 4 tablespoons water
- ½ teaspoon calcium water that comes with the pectin powder

Directions:

1. Combine strawberries and water in a saucepan. Place the saucepan over medium heat.
2. When it starts boiling, turn down the heat to low heat and let it simmer until the berries burst and the juices are released.
3. Stir in calcium water.
4. Combine sugar and pectin powder in a bowl and add into the saucepan. Stir well.
5. Let it cook for about a minute. Turn off the heat.
6. Spoon the jam into 2 sterilized jars. If you want to store it for a long period of time, process the jars in a water bath canner. Make sure to leave a headspace of ¼ inch while canning the jars.
7. If you do not want to process the jars in a water bath canner, you can place the jars in the refrigerator. The jam may last for 3–4 weeks.

Blueberry Frozen Yogurt

Serves: 4

Ingredients:

- ¼ cup granulated sugar
- 6 ounces frozen wild blueberries
- ½ teaspoon lemon zest
- ½ teaspoon vanilla extract
- 2 teaspoons lemon juice
- 1 cup low-fat Greek yogurt

Directions:

1. Mix together blueberries, sugar, lemon juice, vanilla, and lemon zest in a saucepan.
2. Cook the mixture over medium heat until sugar dissolves completely, stirring often.
3. Slightly mash the berries while cooking. Turn off the heat.
4. Transfer the berry mixture into a bowl and cool for a while. Cover the bowl with cling wrap and chill for 3–4 hours.
5. Pour the chilled mixture into a blender and blend until smooth.
6. Add yogurt and blend until well combined.
7. Pour the blended mixture into an ice cream maker and churn the ice cream following the manufacturer's instructions.

8. You can serve now if you want soft serve consistency. For harder yogurt, spoon into a freezer safe container and freeze until use.

Juneberry Jam

Makes 1 jar

Ingredients:
- 3 cups juneberries
- 2 tablespoons water
- 4 tablespoons cane sugar

Directions:
1. Add juneberries, water, and cane sugar into a saucepan. Place the saucepan over medium-high heat. Cook until the berries burst. Stir often. Mash some of them and cook until the jam is thick. Remember the jam will thicken on cooling.
2. Pour the jam into a Mason's jar. When the jam cools, fasten the lid and place in the refrigerator. It can last for 7–8 days.

Mulberry or Blackberry Sorbet

Serves: 8–10

Ingredients:

- ½ cup sugar
- 2 ½ cups red mulberries, discard the green stems
- ½ cup water
- 1 tablespoon cassis or Port wine

Directions:

1. Combine sugar and water in a saucepan. Place the saucepan over medium heat.
2. Stir often until it starts boiling. Turn down the heat to low heat and let it cook for about 3 minutes. Remove from heat and set aside for a while to cool.
3. Place mulberries in a blender. Add warm sugar syrup and blend until smooth.
4. Pour into a bowl.
5. Add port wine and stir. Cover the bowl and place in the refrigerator for about 1 hour.
6. Churn the mixture in an ice cream maker following the manufacturer's directions.
7. Pour into a freezer safe container and freeze for a couple of hours.
8. Scoop into bowls and serve.

Don't hesitate to change the recipes as per your needs and preferences. There is so much more you stand to gain from nature. You will learn about nature's tiny pharmaceutical units, aka edible mushrooms, in the next chapter.

Chapter 6:

Shroomin' Around

Mushrooms are miniature pharmaceutical factories, and of the thousands of mushroom species in nature, our ancestors and modern scientists have identified several dozen that have a unique combination of talents that improve our health. –Paul Stamets

Mushrooms are fungi that usually show up after rains. Chances are you have seen them on rotting wood and logs. You may encounter different species of mushrooms when foraging in the Mountain West region. Some are considered prized possessions in the culinary world, and others have medicinal applications. You will learn about different types of edible mushrooms and tips for identifying them, and recipes to use them in this chapter.

Usually, mushrooms not only taste delicious but are a powerhouse of nutrients as well. Their umami and earthy flavor, combined with all their minerals and nutrients, makes mushrooms an excellent addition to your diet. Most mushrooms are packed with essential nutrients, such as antioxidants, minerals, and vitamins. Regular consumption of mushrooms is thought to stabilize blood sugar levels, improve the strength and functioning of the immune system, and tackle oxidative stress.

Things to Remember

Many experienced foragers will not deal with mushrooms because the risks are too high. Before you start harvesting mushrooms, working with a regional expert or a local forager is essential. The problem with mushrooms is that they're quite small, and the identifying factors are not always easy to distinguish. If you don't look at the mushrooms carefully, you can confuse the poisonous ones with edible ones. In the wild, eating one wrong mushroom can prove fatal. So, if you forage in the Mountain West region, work with an experienced forager before doing it yourself. As explained many times throughout this book, all types of foraging require certainty before handling and eating. Working with mushrooms requires a level of sophistication and expertise beyond some other areas of foraging and therefore it is absolutely crucial to work with an expert each time you are foraging mushrooms in order to evaluate every mushroom you decide to work with.

Also, always carry a field guide and a magnifying glass. When it comes to mushrooms, a magnifying glass is an incredibly helpful identification tool because it enables you to check the spores carefully (without touching). In most cases, the mushroom spores are extremely small and invisible to the naked eye. Checking this is another way to ensure whether you have identified the right mushroom or not. Tools are essential when it comes to foraging! Please investigate what tools are required and recommended for your specific adventure.

You will once again need to carry a basket if you want to harvest mushrooms. They are delicate and fragile and are squished easily. They also start reacting to oxygen after being removed from the growing environment. To ensure the mushrooms don't turn black immediately, you will also need paper bags to keep them safe. The ideal time to gather mushrooms is usually after it rains. Depending on the variety, some mushrooms can also be gathered throughout the year. They prefer wooded and forested areas along with damp and moist regions.

In most Mountain West regions, you will require a permit to pick mushrooms. There is also a limit on the quantity that can be picked for personal consumption and use. Don't forget to carry a small hand spade or trowel with you. This is the best way to carefully dislodge the mushrooms without damaging their structure and without touching them with your skin before you are back home and can consult with your expert.

Edible Mushrooms to Look For

The Mountain West region is home to a variety of edible mushrooms. Again, be sure to follow the suggestions mentioned in the previous section and throughout the guide when it comes to mushrooms. Check and then recheck to ensure you found edible mushrooms and not their poisonous look-alikes. With this in mind, let's look at the different varieties of delicious and nutritious edible mushrooms.

Chicken of the Woods

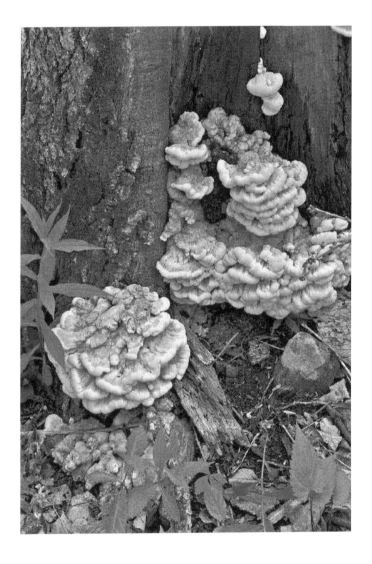

Chicken of the woods mushrooms is also known as the sulfur shelf mushrooms or chicken mushrooms. They are named so because of their typical chicken-like flavor. Because of their taste and texture, these mushrooms are commonly used as a chicken substitute. The scientific name of these mushrooms is *Laetiporus sulphureus*. Identifying and foraging these mushrooms is quite easy due to their size and easy visibility. So, these mushrooms are perfect for foragers of all levels of experience.

Chicken of the woods is among the largest mushrooms. These mushrooms are commonly found in shades of orange and red when young. As they slowly mature, they take on a peach tinge or even turn white. Unlike other mushrooms, these don't have any gills. This factor, coupled with their size and color, makes it quite easy to locate them in the wild. Unlike a typical mushroom, they don't have any stalks and develop in fan-like overlapping clusters or shelves. Since they grow in clusters, it is quite likely that there will be more nearby if you find one. So, don't forget to check the surroundings for a better harvest. Another feature that distinguishes them from typical mushrooms is they don't grow directly out of the soil. Instead, you will find them on the trunks of deciduous trees. These mushrooms are a powerhouse of nutrients and taste incredibly good. They are filled with different anti-inflammatory, anti-bacterial, and antifungal compounds along with Vitamins A and C, potassium, fiber, and antioxidants. While harvesting, opt for the young mushrooms with orange-red caps instead of the mature ones. The mature mushrooms are almost always indigestible and can trigger different allergic reactions too.

Chanterelle

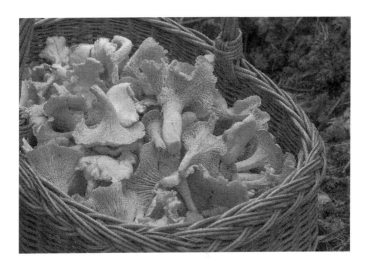

Identifying chanterelles can be straight forward, and they are quite common in the Mountain West region. They are scientifically known as *Cantharellus cibarius*. These mushrooms are a gourmet delight and taste wonderful. They are usually found in hues of bright yellow with a tinge of orange. Their bright color makes them stand out, and thus, foraging can be exciting, especially for those just getting started. (But you still need to check with a local expert before you touch or eat them.)

To identify these mushrooms, carefully check their gills, which will seem as if they are melting away into the stalk. The smell of these mushrooms is almost like that of apricots. The brightly colored cap curls upward toward the edges while the middle portion dips inward. The cap starts to flatten as the mushroom matures. So, the mature mushrooms are usually flat when compared to the curly young ones. These mushrooms are rich in helpful fats, gut-strengthening probiotics, vitamins A, B, C, D, and E, and amino acids. Their mild and slightly fruity flavor makes them a perfect addition to various dishes. Adding these mushrooms will instantly enhance a dish's flavor profile, whether it is a stir-fry, pasta, couscous, or even risotto.

Mountain Morels

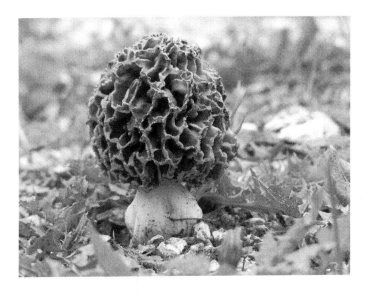

Morel mushrooms are incredibly delicious. They are considered to be a prized possession and a true culinary delight. The scientific name of these popular mushrooms is *Morchella esculenta*. They are characterized by dark brown and oval caps featuring a wavy honeycomb structure. This honeycomb structure is peppered with even darker holes than the rest of the cap. Unlike other mushrooms, they don't have visible gills on the undersurface and are directly connected by the stalks to the hollow caps.

You must remember to carefully check and then recheck whether you have mountain morels on your hand or false morels. Unlike mountain morels, false morels don't have their characteristic intricate honeycomb pattern on the cap. Even though they resemble each other, false morels are incredibly harmful to humans. Don't purely rely on a single identifying factor when it comes to morels or any other mushroom, for that matter, and always check what you've found with a local expert. Mountain morels have white stalks and hollow caps. Both these features are absent in false morels.

During spring, mountain morels are commonly found across Northern America, including the Mountain West region. These mushrooms usually prefer damp and moist places. Therefore, they are found quite close to water bodies. Provided you found edible mountain morels, they do taste delicious and contain various helpful nutrients, such as copper, phosphorus, B-complex vitamins, magnesium, iron, vitamin D, and zinc.

Porcini

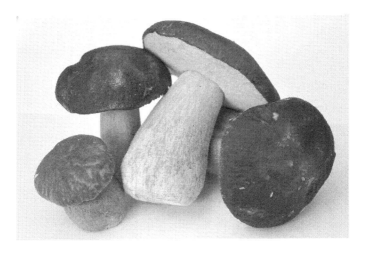

Porcini mushrooms are delicious mushrooms commonly used in French and Italian cuisine. They are also known as king bolete mushrooms and belong to the bolete mushroom family. The scientific name of porcini is *Boletus edulis*. If you love mushroom risotto or pasta, it is quite likely that you have tasted these mushrooms. They have an wonderful earthy aroma and a meaty texture. Combining these factors makes them a common meat substitute in most dishes. They also contain plenty of antioxidants and are a good source of protein and iron.

They resemble a burger placed on a stick. On the underside, these mushrooms have a reddish-brown tinge but can also be found in shades of red, yellow, orange, and white. However, the reddish-brown variant is the most commonly found mushroom in the wild.

They are also characterized by their large cap that is reddish brown too. The cap is usually smooth to touch when the weather is dry. However, it becomes sticky and takes on a cracked appearance when it is wet or moist outside. When you cut into it, the mushroom has pure white flesh. Its stalk is usually yellow or white. It also has tiny white spores on the underside of the cap.

These mushrooms are commonly found in the Mountain West region from June until October. You'll usually find them under birch, pine, and aspen trees. They are delicious added to dishes ranging from broths and pasta to stews, soups, and risotto. If you harvest a bounty of porcini mushrooms and will not be consuming them immediately, dry them and store for later. Once fully dehydrated and stored properly, they will last for a few months. You simply need to rehydrate your mushrooms with stock, broth, or hot water and use as you normally would.

Honey Mushroom

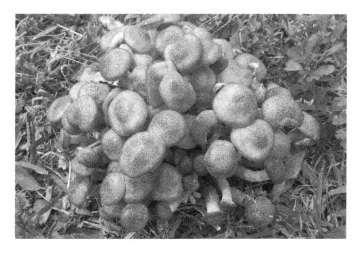

The scientific name of the honey mushroom is *Armillaria mellea*, and it is also known as the honey fungus. These mushrooms are rich in different antioxidants that support and strengthen immune functioning and brain health, have antibiotic properties, and also may regulate blood sugar levels. These delicious and nutritious mushrooms grow in tightly packed clusters and are found on hardwood trees. They are found in the Mountain West region in the United States from late July until November.

The stem of this mushroom is white to begin with and slowly takes on a yellow or yellowish-brown hue as it matures. The stem also has a fine wooly texture. Their cap can be between 5 to 15 cm when fully mature, and their color usually varies from honey-yellow to reddish brown. The area in the center of the cap is usually darker. The flesh itself is white and firm. Initially, the cap is deeply convex, and as it matures, it flattens and develops a wavy margin. You will also notice fine scales on the young caps, especially toward the center. This mushroom is thick but has a tapering base with fairly tough stems. White spores are present on the underside. The gills are crowded and flesh colored. It slowly takes on a yellowish tinge when fully mature. You will also notice rusty spots at this time.

Even though these mushrooms are edible, they are believed to be mildly toxic when eaten raw. Therefore, ensure that you thoroughly cook them before eating. You can cook them like any other mushroom. While foraging for these mushrooms, pick the young ones because they taste the best. It is better to avoid the stems because they are quite chewy and fibrous and don't have much flavor. If the mushroom cap opens up and takes on a brownish color, it is better to avoid it because it can sometimes result in digestive distress.

Lobster Mushroom

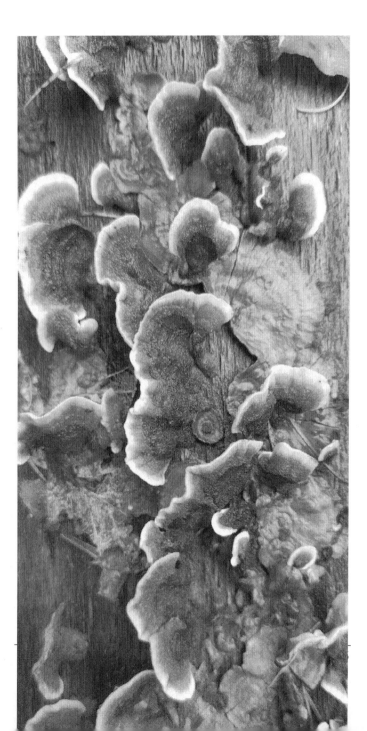

The lobster mushroom is a meaty white mushroom parasitized by a specific fungus known as *Hypomyces lactifluorum*. Because of this parasitic fungus, the host mushroom turns red, and its flavor and textures change. This mold usually attacks only white and large capped mushrooms such as other Russula and Lactarius mushrooms. They have an extremely short shelf-life, but when harvested early and prepared properly, they taste just like lobster! Their color and flavor are why these mushrooms are known as lobster mushrooms. These mushrooms contain essential nutrients, such as vitamin D, phosphorus, zinc, and fiber. A combination of these factors can improve immune functioning, strengthen cardiovascular health, reduce constipation, tackle inflammation and oxidative stress, and promote the production of red blood cells.

These mushrooms are usually found across North America from late July until October and prefer old-growth forests. So, if you are foraging in the Mountain West during late summer and early autumn, keep an eye out for these delicious mushrooms. These mushrooms taste incredible due to their delicate and nutty flavor profile and can be stewed, sauteed, or even deep-fried.

The first identifying factor of these mushrooms is their appearance, their typical bright red-orange hues. The fungus only covers the outer surface of the host mushroom, so the flesh will still be white on the inside. Only harvest those mushrooms that are heavy. If the mushroom is relatively light, it is old and no longer edible. Another factor is their smell. If the mushrooms smell damp or fishy, then avoid them because they are no longer fit for consumption. Some common trees on which you will find them include birch, pine, and other hardwood trees that Russula and Lactarius mushrooms grow on.

Recipes

Mushrooms, indeed, are miniature pharmaceutical factories found in nature. Once you have learned to identify and have successfully harvested them, it is time to learn to incorporate them into different dishes. Use the different recipes in this section to make the most of the mushrooms you have foraged.

Chanterelle and Watercress Puffs

Serves: 8

Ingredients:
- 1.1 pounds chanterelles, trimmed, chopped into chunks
- 14.1 ounces store bought puff pastry
- 2 tablespoons olive oil
- ¼ cup finely chopped, toasted hazelnuts
- salt to taste
- 2 eggs, beaten
- freshly ground pepper to taste

- 14 ounces watercress
- flour to dust
- 2 large cloves garlic, peeled, sliced
- ¼ teaspoon ground nutmeg
- 2 tablespoons fresh orange juice

Directions:

1. Place a pot of water with 2 teaspoons of salt over high heat. When water starts boiling, add watercress and cook for 5 minutes.

2. Drain off in a colander. Press extra moisture from the watercress. Chop watercress into fine pieces.

3. Pour oil into a large pan and let it heat over medium heat. When the oil is hot, add mushrooms and garlic and stir fry for a few minutes until tender.

4. Stir in orange juice and watercress.

5. Add hazelnuts, nutmeg, salt, and pepper and mix well. Turn off the heat. Let it cool completely.

6. Sprinkle some flour on your countertop. If the pastry is not pre-rolled, then roll it into 2 squares with thickness slightly less than ¼ of an inch. If the pastry is pre-rolled, it is generally in a rectangular shape, cut into 2 square shapes, the size of the square will be the breadth of the rectangle.

7. Cut each square into 4 equal squares.
8. Divide the mushroom mixture among the squares, and place it in a triangular shape on one half the squares, along the diagonal, leaving ¼ inch along the borders. Brush the egg all around the edges of the squares. Fold the other half of the square over the filling and press to seal the edges. You will get a triangular shape. Repeat this process with all the squares.
9. Make a couple of small slits on top of the triangles; this is done to release steam while baking. Place triangles on a baking sheet.
10. Preheat the oven to 375° F.
11. Brush egg on top of the puffs.
12. Place the baking sheet in the oven and set the timer for about 20 to 30 minutes or until golden.
13. Cool for a few minutes before serving.

Sautéed Honey Mushroom Caps and Stems

Serves: 4

Ingredients:

- 3-4 clusters of honey mushrooms with their stems
- 2 tablespoons canola oil or any other cooking oil

- salt to taste
- 2 tablespoons unsalted butter
- any other spices or seasoning of your choice

Directions:

1. Separate the stems and caps of the mushrooms. The stems of the mushrooms are to be peeled and the caps trimmed.
2. Pour oil into a large pan and let it heat over high heat. When the oil is hot and slightly smoking, drop the mushroom caps into the pan and mix well.
3. Stir-fry for about 3 minutes. Stir in the mushroom stems and stir-fry for about 3 minutes.
4. Cook until golden brown. Stir now and then. Stir in butter, salt, pepper, and spices if using. Mix well.
5. Serve hot.

Wild Mushroom Bisque

Serves: 3

Ingredients:

- 2 ounces dried edible wild mushrooms of your choice , broken into pieces
- 2 tablespoons unsalted butter, divided

- ½ large yellow or white onion, minced
- salt to taste
- 1–2 tablespoons heavy cream
- pepper to taste
- chopped fresh herbs of your choice to garnish
- 2 ½ cups hot water
- ½ pound fresh bolete mushrooms, minced + extra to garnish
- 3 tablespoons sherry or brandy
- ½ teaspoon dried thyme

Directions:

1. Place mushrooms in a bowl of hot water. Let it re-hydrate for 45–60 minutes.
2. Remove mushrooms with a slotted spoon. Do not discard the soaked water. Chop the mushrooms into fine pieces. Strain the soaked water and keep it aside.
3. Add 1 ½ tablespoons of butter into a soup pot and let it melt over medium heat. When the butter melts, add onion and bolete mushrooms and sauté until light brown.
4. Stir in finely chopped rehydrated mushrooms and stir-fry for a couple of minutes.
5. Stir in thyme, salt, and sherry. Scrape the bottom of the pot to remove any browned bits that may be stuck.

6. Pour the soaked mushroom water into the pot. When the mixture starts boiling, turn down the heat to low heat and simmer for about 20 minutes. Turn off the heat.
7. In the meantime, add ½ tablespoon butter into a small pan. Place the pan over medium heat. When butter melts, add mushroom and stir-fry until brown.
8. Blend half the soup until smooth and pour it back into the soup pot. Mix well and check for the thickness of the soup. If you find it very thick, dilute the soup with some water. If you are adding water, heat the soup after adding water.
9. Add cream and a generous amount of pepper and stir. Serve hot in bowls garnished with the sautéed mushrooms and fresh herbs.

Fresh Porcini or Bolete Julienne

Serves: 8

Ingredients:

- 8 ounces young porcini or any other bolete mushrooms, cleaned, trimmed, cut into ¼ inch thick slices
- 3–4 tablespoons dry white wine
- ⅛ cup garlic greens

- 4 teaspoons all-purpose flour
- ½ cup grated parmesan cheese or grana padano cheese
- ½ teaspoon minced fresh thyme (optional)
- 4 tablespoons cooking oil
- ½ cup diced yellow onion
- 2 tablespoons unsalted butter
- ½ cup sour cream
- ½ cup grated gruyere
- ⅛ teaspoon freshly grated nutmeg

Directions:

1. Preheat the oven to 375° F.
2. Pour 2 tablespoons of oil into a large pan and let it heat over medium-high heat. When the oil is very hot and slightly smoking, add mushrooms and cook until golden brown. Stir occasionally.
3. Transfer the mushrooms into a bowl. Add salt and pepper to taste.
4. Pour remaining oil into the pan and let it heat over medium-low heat.
5. When oil is hot, add onion and cook for a couple of minutes. Stir in the garlic and cook until the onions are soft.
6. Stir in the mushrooms, thyme, and butter. When the butter melts, add flour and nutmeg

and stir. Cook for a minute or so until roux is formed

7. Pour wine into the pan. Scrape the bottom of the pan to remove any browned bits that may be stuck.

8. Add sour cream, gruyere cheese, and parmesan cheese and mix well. Add salt and pepper to taste. Simmer until the cheese melts and you have a thick sauce. Turn off the heat.

9. Spoon the mixture into a baking dish.

10. Place the baking dish in the oven and set the timer for 15 minutes or until brown at a few spots.

11. Remove the baking dish from the oven and let it cool for 5 minutes.

12. Serve.

It's been repeatedly mentioned that nature can offer a bounty of foods that humans need. Another need that humans have met using foraged plants is for medicines, specifically herbs. Herbs not only improve the flavor profile of any dish they are added to but can improve your health. Read on to learn more about some of nature's potentially healing ingredients.

Chapter 7:

Natural Medicine

Herbs are the friend of the physician and the pride of cooks. –
Charlemagne

Foraging is not just restricted to obtaining food for consumption. You can also use this activity to get your hands on nature's pharmacy! Various herbs can be sourced from nature and used for their beneficial properties. Most indigenous people have relied on different herbs to support their physical health and healing. Herbs can even function as a natural insect repellant and a disinfectant.

Things to Remember

One category of wild edibles that can be pretty much gathered throughout the year is herbs. Once you know what you are looking for, identifying and harvesting them can be straightforward. That said, never harvest more than one third of the plant. A wonderful thing about herbs is that they can regrow provided you leave sufficient of the plant behind. Also, the more you harvest, the more the plant will regrow. So, if you find a specific spot of herbs you like or enjoy, make a note of it and revisit it later. You can always come back for a second harvest instead of pillaging the entire area in one go.

You must carry a basket and individual paper bags or covers to store the herbs you have gathered. Herbs are delicate and can be squished easily. In addition to all of the problem-solving techniques you will use to identify potentially edible plants, with herbs you must use your sense of smell (safely, from a distance, without letting the plant touch your skin. If a specific plant does not smell like the intended herb, do not harvest and stay away from it.

Common Herbs to Look For

The different herbs discussed in this section have a variety of medicinal properties. However, they are not a substitute for any medicines you might use, and you must always consult your healthcare provider before adding any herbs to your diet, especially if you are prone to allergies or are taking medications because they can react with one another. Information provided in this section is not intended to diagnose, prescribe, or treat any illness. Always consult a medical professional when treating any illness or injury.

Mallow

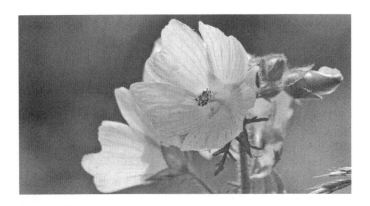

The common mallow's scientific name is *Malva*, which belongs to the *Malvaceae* family, which includes okra and hibiscus. This edible plant has been used as a medicinal remedy for various purposes. The round fruit this plant produces has cheese-like wedges earning this plant its popular nickname cheeseweed.

Though native to northern Africa, Europe, and Asia, they are also found in the Mountain West region within the US. This is a biennial plant that freely branches at the base. It's a low-growing weed with an intricate and fleshy taproot system. The stems can be up to 60 cm long when fully mature.

The flowers can grow individually or in the form of clusters from June until late autumn. The five-petalled flowers are white, pink, or lilac colored. The leaves grow alternatively and are circular or kidney-shaped with toothed and lobed margins. Short hair-like structures are present in the upper and lower leaf areas.

The flowers and leaves of this particular plant offer a variety of medicinal applications, and the essential oil extracted from it may improve overall well-being. It's commonly used as a pain reliever applied topically.

A poultice made using its leaves can be applied on wounds or injured areas to treat the affected region and promote healing. The analgesic properties it offers reduce pain and discomfort. It's used as a topical remedy for headaches. It is considered to strengthen immune functioning and promote internal healing when consumed. It also has anti-inflammatory properties. So, a poultice or gel made from it may help treat sunburn, rashes, insect bites, and large bruises.

It's also used as a remedy for respiratory illnesses and reduce chest congestion. This is once again associated with its anti-inflammatory properties. This plant is also used topically because of their anti-aging benefits that can soothe skin. If you struggle to fall asleep at night, you might sip on a cup of tea brewed using its leaves.

All parts of the correctly identified mallow plant are considered edible. The fruit is commonly used as a substitute for capers, whereas the leaves and flowers can be added to salads. When cooked, the leaves produce a mucus-like substance that can be used as a thickener. The mildly flavored leaves can be used to brew herbal tea.

When boiled in water, a thick mucus-like substance is also released by its roots. This liquid is used as a substitute for egg whites. Also, they are rich in various nutrients, such as vitamins A and C, potassium, selenium, magnesium, and iron. So, mallow is potentially versatile herb.

Nasturtium

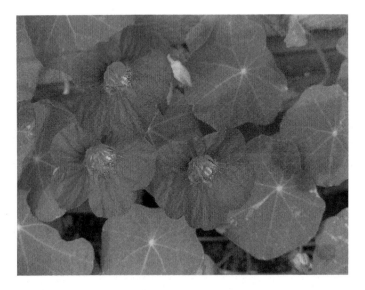

Different species belong to this plant family so their flowers are found in various colors ranging from bright yellow to red and orange. They have big, round leaves with drooping flowers, making them easy to identify. Almost every part of this plant is edible. The leaves have a peppery taste similar to that of mustard greens and watercress. The stems, seeds and roots are also edible and filled with various nutrients.

The flowers and young green leaves of the nasturtium plant are filled with vitamin C. A single ounce of it contains around 130 milligrams of vitamin C. They also contain other essential nutrients, such as manganese, zinc, phosphorus, potassium, calcium, magnesium, and iron. They have a helpful antioxidant known as lutein that may reduce damage caused by free radicals, and also to promote eye and skin health. Nasturtium also contains beta carotene, a form of easily absorbable vitamin A. Due to the high levels of antioxidants in it, nasturtium is commonly used to treat conditions that affect the digestive and respiratory systems. It can also be used topically. The fatty acids in the plant material can act as a natural lubricant and are used in dermatology to treat skin and hair problems. The essential oil extracted from this plant is said to have antibacterial and anti-inflammatory properties that may help with congestion, respiratory infections, colds, and even urinary tract infections when consumed.

If you have ever used microgreens or edible flowers, then nasturtium can be used similarly. The flowers can be added to salads, whereas the leaves can be turned into a pesto or similar preparation. You can also use different parts of this plant to brew herbal tea to receive its nutritional properties. The seeds are often combined with vinegar and other spices and used just like capers, and the mild pepper-like flavor of this plant makes it a helpful substitute for watercress leaves.

Chickweed

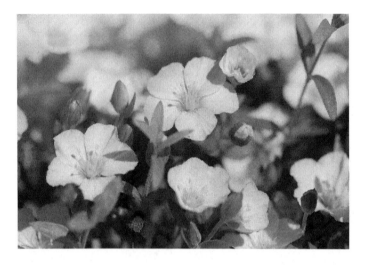

The scientific name of common chickweed is *Cerastium fontanum*. Even though it's considered a pesky weed in most gardens, it is filled with various nutritional benefits and has various medical applications. It doesn't have any specific soil requirements or conditions and, therefore, grows across a variety of habitats, as well as soil types. It is found along the roadsides in cultivated fields, wastelands, and any other terrain you can think of. It is commonly found throughout the United States, including the Mountain West region. So, the next time you head outdoors, you may keep an eye out for this herb, but, again, don't harvest it or any plant in an area that may be contaminated.

These plants grow in an intertwined manner that gives them a unique appearance. They sport small white flowers that start appearing from early spring onwards. The flowers stand out and are quite small and white. They appear in loose branching clusters. Each flower has five petals, and they are all bunched together. The flower stalk also appears slightly hairy.

The stalkless leaves have smooth edges and are usually egg-shaped. The leaves can be up to 2.5 cm long. The leaves on the upper parts of the plant are usually more oblong or lance-shaped than the ones at the bottom. A fully mature chickweed plant can be up to 50 cm tall. The seemingly erect stems usually sprawl on the ground and root at the nodes. The stems are covered with a fine covering of hair-like structures, giving them a fuzzy appearance.

Chickweed contains potentially helpful compounds, including triterpene saponins, vitamin C, flavonoids, and other active plant compounds. Consuming chickweed may support digestive health and is considered to help loosen phlegm or mucus.

The topical application of chickweed may promotes healing due to its anti-inflammatory properties and some traditional Chinese medicine providers may use chickweed to heal infections and wounds.

The leaves, stems, and flowers are the only edible parts of this plant. They can be eaten raw or even added to salads. You can add them to soups and stews, too. Ensure that you opt for tender and young leaves and stems. As they mature, their flavor reduces and becomes tough to chew.

The edible parts of this plant can be crushed and directly applied to irritated skin to tackle inflammation, if you are certain you won't have a sensitivity to it. Chickweed can be consumed as an herbal tea, too.

Ginseng

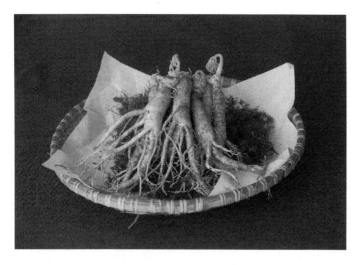

The scientific name of American ginseng is *Panax quinquefolius*. This perennial herb is found across the eastern US, especially under the canopies of deciduous forests. This plant once thrived along the eastern seaboard, but is now endangered in certain areas because of excess harvesting. Ginseng root is incredibly popular because of its potential healing properties. Therefore, before you decide to forage ginseng root in any area, check the local laws and regulations carefully. It is legal to harvest wild ginseng only during a specific season, and these guidelines differ from state to state. If the plant is less than ten years old, it cannot be harvested for export. Usually, American ginseng root can be harvested throughout the month of autumn, but once again, certain licenses are needed. As a rule of thumb, anyone harvesting wild ginseng must not harvest young seedlings, and all mature seeds they come across must be planted.

One of its distinguishing features is the three-pronged five-leaflet presentation of foliage on the mature plant. During the digging season, keep an eye out for red berries. Toward the end of the growing season, the foliage takes on a unique yellowish tinge. If you come across a ginseng plant with only one compound leaf and three leaflets, let it grow because it is still a one-year-old seedling. At this stage, the root of this plant is only about an inch long. Therefore, letting it mature for at least five years is better. This is a deciduous plant, and its leaves usually drop during fall. As the weather warms up during spring, a small rhizome or a neck develops at the root's top. From this bud, new leaves will start sprouting. A fully mature plant can be between 12 to 24 inches tall and usually has over four leaves. Each set of leaves contains five leaflets. The leaflets themselves are around five inches long and have serrated edges. Greenish yellow flowers are produced in clusters during Midsummer, and crimson berries show up a little later.

These plants usually love well-drained and moist soil. They are also commonly confused with Virginia creeper or young Hickory, especially when young. They are predominantly found in the Appalachian region within the United States and the eastern half of North America, ranging from Minnesota to Oklahoma and Georgia in the South, but you may find them in parts of the Mountain West as well.

Ginseng holds a special place with many traditional Chinese medicine providers. Its medicinal benefits are due to two important compounds: ginsenosides and gintonin. It is filled with different antioxidants and is considered to boast a variety of anti-inflammatory properties. Regular consumption of ginseng is considered to reduce inflammation and improve skin health.

Additionally, people who want to improve cognitive functioning and mood, often add some ginseng to their diet. It may also have positive effects on the functioning of the immune system. It is said to improve overall energy levels and tackle fatigue and may regulate blood sugar levels by improving the functioning of the pancreas.

Harvesting this plant takes a little extra effort even after you check all of the local regulations associated with it. You need to carry a shovel or a spade along if you are going to look for ginseng. Slowly start digging a couple of inches away from the base of the stem of this plant. You need to dig to easily work the shovel under the root of the plant and gradually loosen the soil around it. As mentioned, only dig the roots of mature plants and always start digging after the seeds are dark-colored. Please be careful while doing it, and if you notice any seeds, be sure to plant them nearby.

This root can be consumed in different ways. You can either eat it raw or soften by steaming it. It can be steeped in water to brew an herbal tea as well. You can easily incorporate ginseng into soups, stews, and stir-fries. Apart from this, the root can be dried and powdered. The powder can then be incorporated into dishes of your choice.

Goldenseal

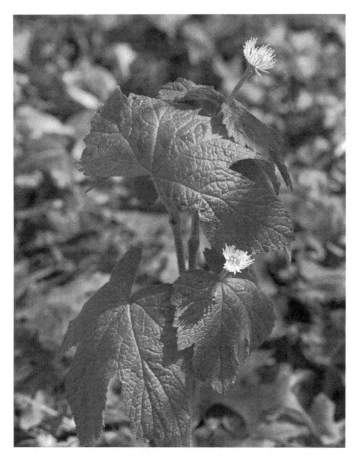

The scientific name of goldenseal is *Hydrastis canadensis*. It belongs to the buttercup family and is commonly found in woodlands. You can often find goldenseal, a perennial herb, in hardwood forests. Foraging this herb is fairly straightforward, provided you know what you want. So, let's learn about its identifying factors. This perennial herb can be up to 20 inches tall and has hairy unbranched stems. The stems usually seem reddish toward the base of the plant and take on a greenish hue toward the upper parts.

This plant sports two types of leaves. The first type consists of small basal leaves withering away when the plant blooms. They are not always found in all plants. The second type of leaves are two-stemmed leaves found on the plant's upper part. The lobed and heart-shaped leaves have serrated margins and an indented center. The leaf margins have fine hair-like structures on the upper and under surfaces. Usually, a solitary flower might appear at the top of the plant, right above the upper leaf. However, all plants don't necessarily flower every year. The flower itself is three-fourths of an inch in diameter when fully bloomed. Around late July, the plant sports clusters of small fruits that resemble raspberries. Each cluster of bright red berries has a short beak and contains ellipsoid black seeds.

This plant has different medicinal applications, and many herbalists use goldenseal to treat skin disorders, digestive troubles and infections of the respiratory tract and can be used as a mouthwash too.

As with every plant mentioned in this guide, ensure that you do not consume too much goldenseal because when consumed in large doses, it overwhelms the system and can result in convulsions in extreme cases. Tea can be brewed using either fresh or dried roots of this plant. It can also be used to make homemade tinctures. Goldenseal should be avoided during pregnancy because it may cause uterine contractions. (Be careful and always check anything with your health care provider.)

Recipes

Well, your job doesn't end after you have identified and possibly gathered different herbs found in the Mountain West. Here are a few preparations to incorporate a variety of herbs into your diet if you'd like.

Mallow Tea

Ingredients:

- 2 teaspoons dried mallow or 8–10 fresh mallow leaves or flowers or mixture of both
- 2 cups water

Directions:

1. Pour water into a saucepan. Add the mallow leaves or flowers or both. Place the saucepan over medium-low heat.
2. When it starts boiling, turn down the heat to low heat and let it simmer for about 10–15 minutes.

3. Strain the tea. You can drink it cold or hot or warm.
4. Don't drink more than 3–4 cups of this tea.
5. You may consider using the tea as a gargle.

Nasturtium Tea

Ingredients:
- 4 cups boiling water
- 2 cups nasturtium flowers and buds

Directions:
1. Put the flowers and buds in a pitcher or jug. Pour boiling water over the flowers.
2. Cover the pitcher and let it infuse for 15 minutes.
3. Strain the tea and use as required.
4. For cold and flu, drink hot or warm tea 2 to 3 times a day.
5. For hair growth, apply the tea to the scalp and massage lightly.
6. Great toner for oily skin.
7. Chewing nasturtium leaves helps boost appetite and helps in digestion.
8. Pour the tea into a spray bottle and spray over the plants to help against insects and bugs.

Herbal Tea with Ginseng

Serves: 5

Ingredients:

- 1 cup dried baby chrysanthemums
- 1/8 cup loosely packed licorice root
- 1 ½ tablespoons rock sugar (optional)
- 1/8 cup loosely packed goji berries
- 1 tablespoon American ginseng
- 5 cups water

Directions:

1. Put the chrysanthemums, licorice root, goji berries, and ginseng in a pot. Pour water into the pot and place it over medium-high heat.
2. When water starts boiling, stir in rock sugar. Keep stirring until sugar melts.
3. Lower the heat and cook covered for about 40–45 minutes. Do not uncover during this cooking process.
4. Turn off the heat and give it a good stir. Strain the mixture and discard the herbs.
5. The tea is ready to serve. You can serve it cold or hot as well.
6. You can drink this tea 1–2 times daily.

There may be instances when you are not immediately utilizing all the foods you have gathered in the wild. What will you do with your edible wild harvest if you are not using it immediately? You will need to store it for later! Read on to learn more.

Chapter 8:

Squirrel It Away

Nature does not hurry, yet everything is accomplished. –Lao Tzu

Until now, you were introduced to information to identify and possibly forage different ingredients in the wild. You were introduced to lists of commonly found greens, nuts and seeds, berries, roots, mushrooms, and herbs in the wild. Take the time needed to thoroughly commit that information to memory, consult with local expert(s), plan your trip including what edible plants you may find plus how to deal with any wild animals you may encounter, all before you go on your foraging adventure. Apart from learning about all this, it is also essential to understand how to enjoy the ingredients you may gather.

Now, let's be practical. There will be instances when you don't want to immediately consume the ingredients, or perhaps the harvest is too big, and you cannot consume it right away. In such instances, learning to preserve can be a good idea. Food preservation is an essential aspect of sustainable living. Whether you are trying to be environmentally conscious, reduce the grocery bill, or simply reduce wastage, food preservation steps into the picture. Food preservation is incredibly simple, and the results will pleasantly surprise you. When done correctly, you can easily increase the shelf life of the ingredients by a couple of weeks or even months in some instances. So, let's learn more about it.

Using Edible Greens

The best thing you can do when it comes to fresh harvested (correctly identified) greens is to consume them immediately. They can be sauteed and stir-fried or added to salads. Depending on how you want to consume them, plenty of options are available. You must understand that greens are a big part of the plant. As soon as they are separated from their roots, they start wilting. Therefore, a simple thing you must do to prolong their shelf-life is to place them in cold water as soon as you can after picking them. This also helps thoroughly clean the greens. This additional step also prolongs their shelf-life and retains their bright green color. In fact, use this suggestion to prolong the shelf-life of greens purchased as well.

Freezing

There are two simple methods for preserving wild greens. The first is to blanch and freeze, and the second is known as freeze-wilting.

When it comes to blanching, bring a pot of water to a rolling boil. If you want, you can add some salt. Place the greens in hot water until they start wilting, and immediately transfer them into a pot of ice-cold water. The shock caused by the temperature change helps the greens retain their natural color. After this, simply place them in bags and keep them in the freezer.

The next option is freeze-wilting. Once the greens are clean, and you have patted them dry with a kitchen towel to get rid of excess moisture, place them in a container or a bag and put it in the freezer. Once they are frozen, remove the bag from the freezer and let the greens thaw at room temperature. Divide the greens into different containers, label them, and refreeze until you need to use them again.

The first method of blanching and freezing usually works for all greens, whereas the second one is especially ideal for flavorful greens. So, watercress, mustard greens, or any other greens that are directly added to a salad or will lose flavor when cooked should be directly frozen, and not blanched first.

Brewing Tea

In the previous chapters, you were introduced to medicinal herbs, their properties, and suggestions about utilizing them. You might have noticed that most herbs can be easily turned into herbal teas. Making it is pretty easy too. The first step is to gather the harvested ingredient and thoroughly clean it. While cleaning, double-check to ensure that you have the right plant on your hand and have not misidentified a poisonous look-alike. Clean it such that there is no debris or dirt in it. Consult with your local expert to be certain, and discard the plant material if you have any doubts. Once you are happy with it, it's time to start brewing the tea.

Start by heating water in a saucepot. As the water comes to boil, add the herbs of your choice. Turn off the heat, place a lid on it, and let it rest for a couple of minutes. Once the water is of the ideal temperature or lukewarm, strain the concoction into a cup and sip. You can always sweeten it with a little honey, maple syrup or sugar. Whenever you make herbal teas, don't forget to taste the herb before brewing. If they are particularly bitter or unpleasant, then sipping a tea made from it will not be easy, even if you sweeten it with honey. Alternatively, you can add other ingredients to flavor it, such as ginger or spices of your choice. Sip on the brew to obtain the benefits associated with it.

Drying

Freezing is not the only option available when extending the shelf life of the foraged greens. Another option available at your disposal is to dry the herbs and store them. This is perfect for any herbs that you have gathered. There are two ways to dry any ingredient of your choice (including even berries and roots).

The first method of drying is known as air drying and the second method involves drying using an oven or a dehydrator. If you decide to air dry the herbs or the greens, you'll first need to thoroughly clean them. Once you know they're clean and free of all dirt and debris, it's time to group them into small bunches. Ensure that around 5 to 10 branches are together. Secure this small bundle using a rubber band or string. The herb bundles need to be placed stem-side up in a paper bag. The end of the paper bag must be secured once again to ensure the herbs are not crushed. Poke a couple of holes in the bag for ventilation, and then hang this bag by the stems in a warm room. Ensure that the room is well-ventilated, or the herbs will not dry. It will take a week or so for the herbs to be fully dry, and as soon as they are brittle to the touch, they are good to be used.

Air drying is effective, but it can take time. You can circumvent the time spent doing this by using a dehydrator or an oven. Place the cleaned ingredients on parchment paper and then in the dehydrator. Within a couple of hours, the ingredients will be fully dry and can be stored. If you are using an oven, you need to line a tray with parchment paper, place the plant material on it, and set the oven to the lowest temperature. You might also need to leave the oven door slightly ajar to ensure better air circulation. Within a couple of hours, the ingredients will be dry. As soon as the ingredients crumble easily or are dry to touch, they are perfect. Store them in airtight containers. These containers can be placed in the freezer as well. Dried herbs can often go for up to one year if stored properly. The dried herbs can then be used just like you have used the fresh ones.

What to Do With Berries

The berries you have foraged don't have to be consumed immediately. You can also store them for later, especially the seasonal varieties. Have you ever purchased berries from a local grocery store in big containers? You carefully get them home, place them in the refrigerator, and then they go bad within a few days! You might not even get an opportunity to eat them! Well, this happens because you may not be storing them properly.

If you want to increase the shelf life of the berries foraged, or even purchased for that matter, here is a simple suggestion. You might try to soak them in a solution made of vinegar and water. When you get the berries, clean them, and dunk them into a solution of water and vinegar.

Fill a large bowl with three cups of water and mix two tablespoons of apple cider vinegar. Ensure the vinegar doesn't have an overwhelming flavor, or the flavor of the berries will be destroyed. You simply need to allow the berries to soak in this mixing job for 5 to 10 minutes. Every couple of minutes, gently stir the berries around. Drain the water and then thoroughly rinse them under running water. Dry the berries and move on to storing them.

To store the clean berries, line a container with paper towels. Place the berries and then place a paper towel on it and put another layer of berries such that the box is packed, but there is a little headspace left. Ensure that you don't tightly seal it; instead, keep the lid slightly open to ensure sufficient space for the moisture to escape. Now, keep it in the refrigerator, and the berries will stay fresh for longer than ever before!

Berries can also be added to pies and desserts of your choice. You can also dehydrate them using the methods discussed in the previous section. Apart from that, you can also turn them into a preserve, jam, or jelly. Making a preserve at home is incredibly simple and hardly requires any ingredients. You simply need some sugar and lemon juice. A simple rule is to add a cup of sugar for every pound of berries you use. Adjust the sugar needed as per your taste and preferences. Once you have washed the berries and removed the stalks, leaves, and other inedible bits, it is time to start. Combine the berries and sugar in a pan and let it rest for two hours, or you can also refrigerate it overnight. Transfer the marinated berries and liquid into a saucepot and let it come to a gentle boil. Keep occasionally stirring to ensure the berries don't burn. After this, add a little lemon juice. Adjust the lemon juice as per the acidity needed to cut through the sweetness or tartness of the fruit you are cooking. Keep cooking until it reaches a slightly jam-like consistency, and you are happy with it. Use this as a pie filling and also spread on bread, spoon over ice cream, or freeze in small batches for later use.

How to Use Roots

When it comes to roots that are foraged, once again, the best suggestion is to use them immediately. However, a wonderful thing about roots and tubers is you can store them too. A simple way to do this is to dry and powder them. To get started, clean the roots and remove any dirt and residue. Once they are clean, pat dry with paper towels or tissues. After this, either air-dry or dehydrate them in an oven or dehydrator. Once the ingredients are fully dry, you must turn them into a powder. Place the dried foods in a blender or food processor and blitz until you have a fine powder! For instance, this works well for the kudzu roots you were introduced to earlier. The powdered root can be used as flour or a thickener. The preservation method will vary depending on how you wish to utilize the root.

Sometimes, you can slice the roots and leave them out to dry. Once dry, you can use them to brew herbal teas at home. As mentioned, the technique used will depend on the ingredient and the purpose for which you want to use them. However, you must always remember to ensure that the dried foods are stored properly. If you are freezing them, ensure that you don't keep thawing and refreezing repeatedly. This alters their texture and will spoil their flavor too. It increases the chances of the ingredients going bad as well.

How to Store Nuts

Using foraged nuts can be a great way to reduce grocery bills; however, a couple of extra steps are needed to ensure that the nuts are stored properly and that they don't go bad. An obvious reason for this step is that the ingredients are exposed to elements for longer. Due to this, they have a little extra moisture built up, which is important to get rid of. If not, the nuts will mold and go bad. Don't worry, because this is an incredibly simple step to follow! As soon as the husks are removed from the nuts, spread them out to dry in a well-ventilated area with plenty of shade. Ensure the nuts and seeds are protected from pests and other critters that might feast on them. Once the nuts are dry, place them in the freezer for 48 hours. This process helps get rid of any other insects, bugs, or worms present in them.

When storing nuts, you have two options. You can store them with or without their shell. If you store with their shells intact, they will stay for longer. However, once you remove the shells and store, it is easier and more convenient to use as and when needed. So, it all boils down to preferences. Place the nuts in airtight containers or bags in the freezer. If the nuts smell or taste stale, it is possible the nuts have gone rancid, and you should discard them because they cannot be salvaged. As long as you follow the suggestions given in this chapter and are careful while handling wild edible foods, you can increase their shelf life and preserve them for later.

Well, nature certainly has a lot to offer. From berries and roots to nuts and seeds and greens, nature can cater to your nutritional needs. Apart from this, foraging is a great way to improve your overall quality of life. Nature can be a healer and spending time in the wild outdoors is nourishing and rejuvenating for your body, mind, and soul. Read on to discover how foraging in nature can be very beneficial to health, whether or not any edible plants are brought home.

Chapter 9:

Nature as a Healer

We must take our children into the wild, introduce them to the plants, and teach them of their connection to the earth. In instilling in our children a respect for plant medicine, we not only care for their tender bodies but help pass along the seeds of a tradition that is as old as human life itself. –Rosemary Gladstar

The modern world we live in is something that our ancestors couldn't have even fathomed in their wildest dreams. Gone are the days when we depended only on hunting and gathering to obtain sustenance. Since the advent of agriculture, the concept of gathering and foraging foods in the wild has started to fade away from regular human culture. Even though it is prevalent in some parts of the world, it is not as prevalent as it once was. However, it has steadily gained popularity in the last couple of years.

In recent times, more and more people are realizing how far they have drifted apart from their roots and nature. Open any newspaper and you will find articles and reports about a steadily increasing global concern, environmental pollution. Whether it is the increasing levels of greenhouse gasses or the steadily increasing carbon footprint, we can take steps toward the solution.

Instead of viewing nature as something to consume, you may come to understand that nature is a nurturer, and that spending time in nature can be healing.

To that end, foraging can be a simple yet effective means to increase the time spent in nature and reconnect with it. You are improving the overall quality of life by being out in nature and look for potential foods that grow naturally in the wild. By spending some time in the great outdoors, you get a chance to reconnect with your roots and understand more about the ecosystem. Here are all the different ways foraging can be a great way to heal your body, mind, and soul.

Stress Relief

How would you feel after spending a day in the park or the local woods? Probably relaxed, serene, and rejuvenated. Nature is one of the best stress relievers you can come across. This is an incredible benefit associated with foraging.

Most of us often want to feel more connected to nature and the pleasant feelings it evokes in us. And even though we have made significant progress as a species, oftentimes those advancements can impede upon our happiness.

Chronic stress reduces our productivity and the overall quality of our life, and can contribute to variety of health problems. It affects not only your mental health but physical and emotional well-being, too. For instance, being constantly stressed increases the risk of digestive problems, becomes a source of constant headaches, and prevents good sleep at night.

When you start foraging, you are automatically required to spend more time outdoors. You are spending more time in nature away from all the things that caused your stress. At times, the best means to deal with stress is a simple change of environment. Foraging enables you to disconnect from the hustle and bustle of daily life and, instead, engage in the serene beauty of nature.

More Pleasant Feelings

Previously, it was mentioned that modern living has become a source of chronic stress. The good news is that you can replace these feelings with all things desirable once you start foraging. Nature can be nurturing. Whenever you are overwhelmed by a specific emotion, your mind fixates on it. It keeps thinking thoughts that focus on the said emotions, or keeps replaying circumstances or happenings that further intensify the said emotion. Due to this, you will be consumed by the said emotion. Unfortunately, not all emotions are pleasant, and some are downright unhelpful.

For instance, fixating on anger, sorrow, fear, stress, or regret is not going to do you much good. It may also steal the calm and happiness you have, and it can be difficult to stop the fixating.

One way of working with unhelpful emotions is to distract your mind. When you consciously distract yourself by doing something else or engaging in another activity, your mind is forced to shift gears too. This is where foraging steps into the picture. When you are in the wild outdoors, you must consciously focus on your actions and engage all your senses. When you are thoroughly engaged in the activity, you don't have time to focus on unhelpful emotions. You are problem solving, engaged in critical thinking, and being resourceful. So, in a way, spending time in nature makes room for positive and pleasant feelings.

Natural Healing

Japanese forest bathing, also known as "Shinrin-Yoku," which roughly translates to "Taking in the forest atmosphere," Norwegian forest living, known as "Friluftsliv," and the traditions of many native and Indigenous cultures around the world all center around immersing oneself in nature, which can offer a much-needed eco-antidote to individuals who feel burnt out, while giving people a chance to reconnect with nature and protect it. A variety of cultures across the world have always known the importance of spending time connecting with nature.

Consciously spending time in the wonderful outdoors can be a great way to heal your body, mind, and soul.

Better Immunity

The quality of the air that we breathe is important. Not just because we obtain oxygen from it but because we are exposed to various pollutants these days. When you breathe fresh air while foraging, you breathe in the airborne chemicals released by plants known as phytocides. These phytocides are naturally blessed with antibacterial and antifungal qualities that plants utilize to tackle diseases and illnesses. You are also automatically obtaining these helpful properties when breathing in these chemicals. Your immune functioning improves when you are regularly exposed to natural and fresh air while foraging. A better and stronger immune system automatically reduces your susceptibility to illnesses. After all, health is wealth!

Another wonderful benefit of spending some time outdoors is that this can stabilize your blood pressure levels. High blood pressure is a silent killer and a steadily increasing global health concern. Unfortunately, it is worsened by constant exposure to stress. When stressed, a chemical known as cortisol is produced in the body. This is responsible for our fight-or-flight instinct. This is the same instinct that's triggered when faced with danger. Since the brain cannot distinguish between actual physical danger and mental stress, this response is triggered. When it is only a temporary response, it gives the needed strength or power to escape a potentially life-threatening situation. It is characterized by increased heart rate and blood pressure, reduced energy to non-vital organs, and a burst of energy. However, your blood pressure is steadily elevated if you are constantly in this state. This has serious repercussions, especially on the health of vital organs. Stress harms your body from the inside out. So, start spending more time outdoors reconnecting with nature to help to improve your health and immunity.

Improve Gut Health

Did you know that your gut is home to millions of bacteria known as the gut microbiome? Don't get scared reading the word bacteria! The gut microbiome is extremely helpful and is needed for the digestive system's smooth functioning. Your overall health is compromised if there is any imbalance in the gut microbiome. In the previous section, it was mentioned that foraging is a great way to strengthen your immune system. Did you know that a part of this immune functioning is associated with the balance and health of the gut microbiome? So, you can improve your overall health by taking care of the gut microbiome.

As with any other living creature, the gut microbiome requires nutrition. They get this from the food you consume. A wonderful thing about eating more plants is that they can strengthen the functioning of the gut microbiome. They function effectively and efficiently by giving them the necessary nutrients. A healthy gut microbiome ensures your body gets the nutrition from the food consumed.

Satisfies Our Needs

As mentioned previously, our ancestors were predominantly hunters and gatherers and depended on items they could gather from their surroundings for sustenance. In a way, these behaviors are likely embedded into our DNA and cannot be separated from our personalities. Unfortunately, the modern world has removed us far from the natural world, and so our persistent basic need to gather and explore is often satisfied at the mall or online. The good news is that you can automatically fix the situation by foraging. When you are foraging, it helps satisfy the deep-seated need for gathering and exploring. You will also notice that you get excited when you correctly identify a plant, regardless of whether it is edible or not. Biting into the first luscious berry (you correctly identified) is a thrilling experience. So, it is not only exciting but also caters to your psychological needs.

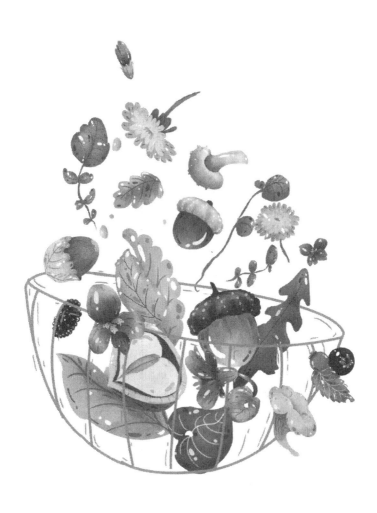

Conclusion

Look deep into nature, and then you will understand everything better. –Albert Einstein

Foraging is not a new activity and is as old as human history on earth. It goes back to the dawn of civilization. Our prehistoric ancestors relied wholly on all foods found in nature for sustenance. With all the developments humans have made and our progress, we have slowly distanced from foraging. Due to this, most of us have also lost touch with Mother Nature. The good news is that all this can be immediately fixed with foraging. Foraging is extremely beneficial, regardless of whether you want to learn more about your local ecosystem or live sustainably and spend more time in the wild outdoors. Unsurprisingly, it is slowly regaining its lost popularity.

This book will act as your guide and introduce you to aspects involved in foraging in the Mountain West region of the United States. From understanding what foraging means and the benefits it offers to becoming an ethical forager and learning the laws and regulations involved, you were introduced to the basics of foraging. You were also introduced to different types of edible foods you might find in the wild. From greens and weeds to flowers, nuts and seeds, fruits, and mushrooms, there is a lot you can identify from your immediate surroundings. However, before you can do that, spend the time needed to familiarize yourself with the different characteristics of plants and how to identify them. Use this information here as a learning tool to help you work effectively with the local expert(s) that you consult.

This book introduced you to different medicinal herbs and their uses. Apart from this, you were also introduced to recipes using the wild ingredients foraged. Using these recipes, you can truly enjoy and honor the delicious foods you foraged. After all, it is not just about spending hours together looking for and harvesting wild foods. Honoring nature's bounty and enjoying it is also important to becoming a forager. As long as you are willing to commit to learning and applying all that you have learned, including working with local experts, you can become an excellent ethical forager!

Foraging not only offers a variety of benefits but is a truly enjoyable activity, too. It gives you a chance to get out of the hectic city life and instead, connect with nature and spend some time outdoors. Once you do this, you will want to do it again. It will soon become a part of sustainable living and allow you to explore new places. You can also breathe fresh air, experience bright sunshine, and exercise. It is a fun bonding activity for not just family but friends as well. You get to try new foods and flavor combinations while obtaining the needed nutrients. Foraging teaches you to learn more about the ecosystem around and feel more connected to it. Also, you can obtain all these benefits with relative ease as long as you plan well and use patience.

The act of foraging includes bending, reaching, walking, grasping, and using our eyes to scan open spaces. We use our brains to problem solve, and we build focus, patience, and determination. All of these elements can be incredibly helpful for our bodies and minds. Even if we don't bring home any food, we've done a lot of good for ourselves. As with all exercise and movement, please make sure you are fit for the task and be prepared with appropriate gear and tools. Please work with your medical provider to determine if trail hiking and outdoor adventure is appropriate for you based on your unique health needs.

By following the information given in this book, you can start foraging wild edibles in the Mountain West region. Don't forget to try different recipes to make the most of the harvested ingredients. After all, foraging is not just about collecting ingredients but learning to honor and enjoy them too. I believe you can rekindle and strengthen your bond with nature and improve the overall quality of your life by foraging!

So, what are you waiting for? Before you start foraging, I have a small favor to ask. Can you please spare a few minutes and leave a review for this book if you enjoyed reading it and found it helpful? Others interested in foraging will benefit from your feedback and insights!

Thank you and all the best!

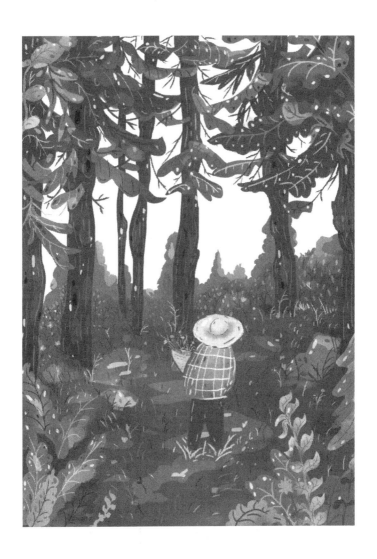

References

Ballard, L. (2018, November 14). Forage wild nuts for your holiday feast. *Cool Green Science.* https://blog.nature.org/science/2018/11/14/f orage-wild-nuts-for-your-

Colleen. (n.d.). Forage archives. *Grow Forage Cook Ferment.* https://www.growforagecookferment.com/for age/

Douglas, J. (2021, May 6). Ethical foraging-responsibility and reciprocity. *Organic Growers School.* https://organicgrowersschool.org/ethical-foraging-responsibility-

Foraging guidelines. (n.d.). Woodland Trust. https://www.woodlandtrust.org.uk/visiting-woods/things-to-do/foraging/foraging-guidelines/

Gardiner, B. (2021, February 14). Nine basic principles of ethical wildcrafting for beginners - the outdoor apothecary. *The Outdoor Apothecary.* https://www.outdoorapothecary.com/ethical-wildcrafting/

Lanier, K. (2017, September 11). Three tips for collecting wild seeds and preserving plant diversity. *Hobby Farms.* https://www.hobbyfarms.com/collecting-wild-seeds/

Linnekin, B. J. (2018, January 9). The case for legal foraging in America's national parks. *The Counter.* https://thecounter.org/the-case-for-legalizing-foraging-in-national-parks/

Responsible foraging guidelines. (n.d.). Colorado Parks and Wildlife. *https://cpw.state.co.us/aboutus/Pages/RulesRegs.aspx*

Universal edibility test: How to test a wild plant's edibility. (2021, November 6). MasterClass. https://www.masterclass.com/articles/universal-edibility-test

Image References

AmatusSamiTahera. (2020, July 7). *Carraway seeds* [Image]. Pixabay. https://pixabay.com/photos/cumin-white-cumin-herbs-ayurveda-5377177/

angelstar. (2014, September 15). *Nasturtium* [Image]. Pixabay. https://pixabay.com/photos/nasturtium-red-flowers-blossom-444387/

Barbroforsberg. (2016, February 12). *Chanterelle* [Image]. Pixabay. https://pixabay.com/photos/fungus-mushroom-sponge-basket-1194380/

Bru-nO. (2020, July 3). *Wild black cherry* [Image]. Pixabay. https://pixabay.com/photos/cherries-wild-cherries-fruit-5363587/

ChiemSeherin. (2018, July 20). *Blueberries* [Image]. Pixabay. https://pixabay.com/photos/blueberries-fruits-berries-food-3548239/

Eiermann, G. (2021, June 26). *Juneberries* [Image]. Unsplash. https://unsplash.com/photos/HWCWK1c63VU

Haerer, J. (2017, April 12). *Goldenseal* [Image]. Pixabay. https://pixabay.com/photos/goldenseal-wildflower-flower-2225968/

Haerer, J. (2017, August 20). *Amaranth seeds* [Image]. Pixabay. https://pixabay.com/photos/amaranth-seed-food-plant-nature-2662885/

Haerer, J. (2020, April 18). *Sassafras* [Image]. Unsplash. https://unsplash.com/photos/cwyg7IG23J8

Hermann, S., & Richter, F. (2016, June 21). *Mallow* [Image]. Pixabay. https://pixabay.com/photos/sigmars-root-mallow-rose-mallow-1468240/

Hermann, S., & Richter, F. (2018, May 7). *Dandelions* [Image]. Pixabay. https://pixabay.com/photos/dandelion-meadow-dandelion-meadow-3381676/

Hiltula, E. (2022, August 10). *Butternuts* [Image]. iStockphoto.com. https://www.istockphoto.com/photo/juglans-cinerea-butternut-gm1413782506-462737107?clarity=false

Hondow, B. (2014, November 7). *Honey mushroom* [Image]. Pixabay. https://pixabay.com/photos/honey-fungus-fungus-fungi-517397/

JamesDeMers. (2012, October 1). *Black walnuts* [Image]. Pixabay. https://pixabay.com/photos/juglans-nigra-eastern-black-walnut-58548/

kellyclampitt. (2019, February 16). *Chicken of the woods* [Image]. Pixabay. https://pixabay.com/photos/fungi-chicken-of-the-woods-mushroom-2069479/

LaBar, M. (2016, August 1). *Hickory nuts* [Image]. Pixabay. https://pixabay.com/photos/nut-pecan-husk-carya-illinoinensis-1550019/

LoggaWiggler. (2011, June 18). *Wild strawberry* [Image]. Pixabay. https://pixabay.com/photos/strawberry-wild-strawberry-red-7649/

MacDonald, B. (2016, August 10). *Staghorn sumac* [Image]. Pixabay. https://pixabay.com/photos/staghorn-sumac-rhus-typhina-1579339/

Macou, J. (2015, November 30). *Persimmons* [Image]. Pixabay. https://pixabay.com/photos/fruit-khaki-fall-persimmon-1065727/

mariastone. (2015, July 8). *Kudzu flower* [Image]. Pixabay. https://pixabay.com/photos/kudzu-flower-japanese-arrowroot-831489/

Meyer, A. (2016, July 13). *Pokeweed* [Image]. Pixabay. https://pixabay.com/photos/pokeweed-asian-pokeweed-blossom-5400622/

Meyer, A. (2022, May 18). *Chickweed* [Image]. Pixabay. https://pixabay.com/photos/mountain-chickweed-arenaria-montana-7204951/

NickyPe. (2019, September 24). *Burdock plant* [Image]. Pixabay. https://pixabay.com/photos/burdock-wild-plant-nature-4497755/

pasja1000. (2018, September 16). *Acorns* [Image]. Pixabay.

https://cdn.pixabay.com/photo/2018/09/16/
20/37/branch-3682386_960_720.jpg

pasja1000. (2018, July 7). *Day lillies* [Image]. Pixabay. https://pixabay.com/photos/lily-orange-daylily-blossomed-5378706/

Pixamio. (2022, June 28). *Wild garlic* [Image]. Pixabay. https://pixabay.com/photos/garlic-wild-garlic-pink-flower-7288422/

Reichelt, M. (2021, Dec 5). *Wild millet seeds* [Image]. Pixabay. https://pixabay.com/photos/millet-grain-wild-grasses-ear-6841396/

Roosink, M. (2014, November 12). *Cattail* [Image]. Pixabay. https://pixabay.com/photos/cattail-loosestrife-stinky-cigar-526000/

Romero, G. A. (2019, May 2). *Red mulberry* [Image]. Pixabay. https://pixabay.com/photos/mora-mulberry-fruits-berry-red-4168076/

Ruigrok van de Werve, K. (2021, November 28). *Lobster mushroom* [Image]. Unsplash. https://unsplash.com/photos/1vOk2_CM8YM

sergei_spas. (2022, August 28). *Red chokecherry* [Image]. Pixabay. https://pixabay.com/photos/berries-bird-cherry-virgin-red-tree-7414212/

Seven75. (2021, February 03). *Watercress* [Image]. iStockphoto.com

https://www.istockphoto.com/photo/nasturtiu
m-officinale-plants-close-up-gm1299255266-
391934902?phrase=watercress

Singhal, N. (2016, July 29). *Dooryard violet* [Image].
Unsplash.
https://unsplash.com/photos/hrlPhAZLyN8

Strauß, J. (2016, April 19). *Mountain morels* [Image].
Pixabay. https://pixabay.com/photos/morel-
morkel-mushroom-1336524/

sunnysun0804. (2015, December 22). *Hazelnuts* [Image].
Pixabay.
https://pixabay.com/photos/hazelnut-nut-
protein-1098181/

szjeno09190. (2015, September 2). *Porcini* [Image].
Pixabay.
**https://pixabay.com/photos/mushroom-
porcini-mushrooms-forest-913499/**

Vacchiano, M. (2016, January 23). *Caraway* [Image].
iStockphoto.
**https://www.istockphoto.com/photo/caru
m-carvi-common-names-caraway-meridian-
fennel-gm505407382-
83667459?phrase=caraway%20flower**

whaltns17. (2018, May 16). *Ginseng* [Image]. Pixabay.
https://pixabay.com/photos/ginseng-
medicine-3404958/

WikimediaImages. (2015, July 31). *Plantain* [Image]. Pixabay. https://pixabay.com/photos/plantago-lanceolata-english-plantain-846539/

Made in the USA
Columbia, SC
16 January 2023

10454353R00104